Transcranial Magnetic Stimulation

Transcranial Magnetic Stimulation
A Neurochronometrics of Mind

Vincent Walsh and Alvaro Pascual-Leone

A BRADFORD BOOK

The MIT Press
Cambridge, Massachusetts
London, England

This book was set in Bembo by Interactive Composition Corporation and was printed and bound in the United States of America.

Library of Congress Cataloging-in-Publication Data

Walsh, Vincent, 1961–
    Transcranial magnetic stimulation : a neurochronometrics of mind / Vincent Walsh and
    Alvaro Pascual-Leone.
        p. ; cm.
    "A Bradford book."
    Includes bibliographical references and index.
    ISBN 0-262-23228-6 (hc : alk. paper)
    1. Magnetic brain stimulation. I. Pascual-Leone, Alvaro. II. Title.
    [DNLM: 1. Brain—physiopathology. 2. Magnetics—diagnostic use.
    3. Cognition—physiology. 4. Diagnostic Imaging—methods. 5. Neuropsychology—methods.
    WL 141 W227t 2003]
    RC386.6.M32 W357   2003
    616.89'13—dc21
                                                                    2002035063

10 9 8 7 6 5 4 3 2 1

To Berndt-Ulrich Meyer, Simone Röricht, Marty Szuba, María Dolores Catalá, and Teresa García

Nicht nichts
ohne dich
aber nicht dasselbe.

(Not nothing
without you
but not the same)

Ohne Dich
—Erich Fried (1979)

Contents

FOREWORD: DRAWN TO NEUROMAGNETISM   ix
by Stephen M. Kosslyn

PREFACE: A MAGNETIC MANIFESTO   xv

ACKNOWLEDGMENTS   xix

1   INTRODUCTION: COGNITIVE RESOLUTION   1

2   MAGNETS AND MINDS IN HISTORY   11

3   THE NUTS AND BOLTS OF TMS   39

4   CREATING VIRTUAL PATIENTS: A GUIDE TO MECHANISM
       AND METHODOLOGY   65

5   REAL-TIME NEUROPSYCHOLOGY: SINGLE-PULSE TMS   95

6   DYNAMIC NEUROPSYCHOLOGY: REPETITIVE-PULSE TMS   127

7   The Self-Engineering Brain   163

8   Can I Borrow Your Illness?   199

9   Converging Methodologies: A Meeting of
      Mind's Maps   219

References   231

Name Index   281

Subject Index   289

Cognitive neuroscience is founded on the idea that "the mind is what the brain does." This field is the latest chapter in the centuries-old effort to understand the nature of mental functions such as memory, perception, language, and reasoning. Cognitive neuroscience emerged from two kinds of developments, conceptual and methodological.

First, conceptual advances have helped us to formulate new ways to ask questions about the relation between the mind and brain. These developments grew out of the computer metaphor that characterized cognitive psychology. As originally conceived, this metaphor rested on the idea that the mind is like a computer program, which can be understood independently of the hardware on which it runs. This perspective explicitly marginalized facts about the brain, which were considered largely irrelevant for understanding the mind. This view made pragmatic sense when not much was known about the brain, but began to be eroded as increasing numbers of facts about brain function emerged from the neurologists' clinics and the neurophysiologists' laboratories. Researchers came to realize that the brain is not a general purpose computer, designed to run any program; rather, it evolved in a specific time and place, and its function grows in large part out of its structure. The relation between structure and function became increasingly clear as relatively self-contained systems, such as the retina, were studied in detail.

The shift from the computer metaphor to a brain-based approach reached a tipping point in the mid-1980s, when neural network models came into vogue (in particular, after publication of the volumes edited by David Rumelhart and James McClelland, e.g., in 1986). These models not only conflated structure and process, which seemed so clearly distinct when viewed through the lens of the computer metaphor, but also relied explicitly on the notion that facts about the brain are indeed relevant for understanding the mind.

Although the original neural network models consisted of single networks, it wasn't long before researchers learned that complex tasks require complex processing, and such processing often requires sets of neural networks operating in concert. Thus, one sort of theory that emerged in cognitive neuroscience posits sets of subsystems that work together to accomplish a task. These theories were often guided (either formally or informally) by "computational analyses" of the task at hand. That is, researchers asked what they would need to do in order to build a machine that exhibits specific types of behavior. In particular, David Marr (1982) and Herbert Simon (1981) both offered ways to develop theories of the sorts of processing that might be invoked when one performs a specific task. In both cases, they emphasized the role of the goal, the information available to achieve the goal, and the constraints on ways in which that information can be used. Marr stressed the importance of analyzing *what* must be computed as distinct from *how* computations proceed. Simon stressed that the nature of the task can dictate much of the underlying processing, just as the grains of sand on a beach can determine the path taken by an ant as it makes its way back to its hill. Both theorists stressed that complex tasks can only be achieved by a strategy of divide-and-conquer, solving a host of relatively simple problems that underlie the task in question.

For example, consider the task of visually identifying objects. A necessary first step is to segregate figure from ground, to select a shape that might correspond to an object. Considering the information that is available to accomplish this goal, researchers quickly realized that one way to proceed is to delineate an object's edges. Edges in turn are often signaled by sharp changes in luminance that are present at several levels of scale (and thus aren't simply texture on a surface).

In this case, the constraints might require that points of sharp change must be contiguous, defining a curve.

For present purposes, the most important aspect of task analyses is that they lead one to break processing down into separate components. These separate processes—such as one that detects edges with the goal of defining figure versus ground—work together to accomplish a task. For example, simply detecting edges is not a reliable way to isolate objects, if only because objects are often partially obscured by other objects. Thus, other processes—such as those that "grow" common regions of similar color and texture or that group points that are similar distances from the viewer—should work together with processes that detect edges. Moreover, these processes are the prelude to other processes that compare input to information stored in memory, which in turn lead to yet other processes that use this information in various ways (e.g., in naming).

Theories of processing systems invited other researchers to ask whether the brain in fact respects the hypothesized distinctions, and is organized into processing subsystems as posited by the theory. This conceptual advance was crucial in the development of cognitive neuroscience, but was not itself sufficient: Although one must know how to ask questions before being in a position to answer them, the mere fact that questions can be posed does not imply that the means are available to address them. Thus, it was a happy coincidence that as researchers began to think of the brain in terms of complex sets of neural networks they were also provided with new methodologies for testing such theories. In particular, first positron emission tomography (PET) and then functional magnetic resonance imaging (fMRI) allowed researchers to track activity in the awake, behaving human brain. These techniques are wonderfully concrete, and can localize activity far more accurately than was previously possible. In fact, the spatial resolution of these techniques appears about right for testing theories of processing subsystems.

However, shortly after fMRI became widely used, one of its drawbacks became glaringly obvious: This and related techniques only establish *correlations* between performing a task and activity in certain brain areas. As has become all too evident, different researchers often find different results when using the "same" task. What on the face of things seem to be details in how a task is designed can make a big difference in which areas are activated. However, one issue is whether the areas that are activated in some studies but not others play the same role as those that are consistently activated. Some of these areas that are not consistently activated could be "just along for the ride," activated by connections from other areas or indirectly affected by remote activity elsewhere in the brain. That is, at least some of the activated areas could play no causal role in performing the task.

If a brain area plays a causal role in performing a task, then performance of that task should be impaired if that brain area is damaged. This logic has guided the traditional method of testing theories of the organization of processing systems, which requires finding patients who have suffered brain damage and thereafter exhibit selective deficits. However, such damage is rarely precisely localized in the brain and rarely has highly circumscribed effects. Moreover, the precise locus of most forms of brain damage (typically following a stroke) depends on the brain's vasculature, and thus not all parts of the brain are equally likely to be damaged—which means that some theories will be particularly difficult to test.

Enter transcranial magnetic stimulation (TMS). As Walsh and Pascual-Leone so nicely illustrate in the present volume, one critical virtue of this technique is that it can establish whether specific brain areas play a *causal* role in specific types of processing. By temporarily impairing the functioning of specific patches of cortex, researchers can discover whether the processes accomplished by those neurons do in fact contribute to a specific type of performance. Moreover, the same people can be used both in the experimental condition and the control condition, thereby controlling for a large number of variables (e.g., individual differences in brain organization) that bedevil traditional research with brain-damaged patients. Furthermore, not only can TMS disrupt processing, with appropriate pulse sequences it might also be able to facilitate it. If so, this property has the potential of allowing researchers to sidestep a perennial problem in research with brain-damaged patients: More difficult tasks are proportionally more difficult for them to accomplish. The simple fact that their brains are damaged slows them down, and makes hard tasks harder. Thus, deficits in performance can reflect general difficulties in addition to disruption of specific processes. TMS not only has much more focal effects than brain damage, but also with appropriate parameter values it might be able to boost the relative performance of an area. If this early promise comes to fruition, TMS will thereby have the potential to facilitate specific processing, and to do so only for the specific processes implemented in a particular brain location.

It is difficult to underestimate the importance of being able to demonstrate a causal relation between specific neural activity and performance. In fact, TMS can play a key role in grounding theories of cognitive function in general. Let me explain. Chomsky (1967) discussed three ways we can evaluate theories. First, the weakest form of adequacy consists of a theory's being able to account for a set of data. In linguistics, theories of grammar that have such *observational adequacy* can account for people's intuitions about which sentences are grammatical and which are not. More generally, a theory that is adequate in this way can predict the observed results, be they behavior (response times, error rates, judgments) or patterns of neural activation.

Second, a slightly stronger sort of adequacy requires that a theory can account for the structure within the corpus of data. For example, a theory of grammar would have such *descriptive adequacy* if it could explain how the sentence "John kicked the ball" is related to "The ball was kicked by John." In Chomsky's early theory, a single "kernel" produced both utterances, after being transformed to produce the passive in the second case. More generally, a theory that is adequate in this way can predict which tasks will rely on common underlying processing and which will draw on distinct processes. Such a theory would explain, for example, patterns of individual differences in behavior—why people who can perform one task well will tend to perform well certain other tasks (but not all tasks in general).

Third, the strongest sort of adequacy strikes to the heart of explaining why processing occurs as it does. If a theory has *explanatory adequacy*, it can justify its principles by appeal to other sorts of considerations than the mere fact that the theory accounts for data—or even the patterns in data. If the theorist just sticks with one sort of data, a problem arises: How does one know whether the data that motivated the theory in the first place aren't similar to the "new" data being explained? That is, nobody is impressed by theories that are formulated post hoc, made up to explain specific data. But if the data that were not considered initially are in fact related to those that were initially considered, why should it be surprising that they can also be explained by the theory? The key is to have an "ulterior motive," a separate set of considerations that justify the theory. In the case of language, one such consideration is the ability to learn language. More generally, facts about the brain can play this role for cognitive theories. For example, if the theory posits two distinct processes, this theory gains credibility if researchers show that different parts of the brain implement each process. TMS is a powerful tool for accomplishing this goal. Moreover, TMS can document temporal relations among specific brain processes, which can provide evidence for theories of processing that posit stages or other sequential processing. TMS is a way to ground theories of cognition, not only by showing that activity in brain areas is correlated with distinct processes, but to establish a causal connection between specific types of brain activity and specific cognitive processes.

One strength of TMS is its relative specificity; it can be directed toward a relatively small patch of cortical real estate. However, this strength is also a potential drawback: How does one know where to aim? Ideally, researchers can perform neuroimaging with the same participants, and thereby identify brain regions that are active for a given participant during a particular task. TMS would then be directed toward those specific areas for that specific person. Thus, TMS is not a replacement for neuroimaging, but rather complements it. Using the two tools together provides much more information than would be possible with either alone.

Vincent Walsh and Alvaro Pascual-Leone have written a marvelous overview of what TMS is, what it has revealed so far, and what it could conceivably lead to in the future. This book is as entertaining as it is informative; it presents numerous examples of creative uses of the technique, and is sure to inspire other researchers to adopt this powerful tool. As so beautifully illustrated here, TMS can be used to good end in our continuing quest to understand the mind and its relation to the brain.

Stephen M. Kosslyn

The aim of this book is to promote transcranial magnetic stimulation (TMS) into the mainstream of cognitive neuropsychology. The principal belief behind this book is that the use of TMS to induce virtual lesions can lead to new discoveries about cortical functions, discoveries that cannot be made using other techniques. The virtual-lesion methodology we describe can produce virtual patients with unique patterns of "lesions" and deficits in space and time, and it therefore operates in a new problem space not previously accessible to neuropsychology. The book is not intended to be a technical manual; it is intended to present an insight into a new way of approaching behavioral questions in the cognitive neurosciences. One measure of the accuracy of our aim will be the degree to which the findings of TMS studies are seen to influence neuropsychological theories. Another measure will be the integration of TMS with neuroimaging techniques such as functional magnetic resonance imaging (fMRI), positron emission tomography (PET), magnetoencephalography (MEG), and electroencephalography (EEG). To some extent, both of these processes have begun, but there is still a long way to go, and in our view progress has been slower than it should have been. A remarkable study in 1989 by Amassian and colleagues demonstrated clearly how TMS could be used to test a psychological model and to offer an analysis in both psychological and physiological terms. However, five years elapsed before another laboratory addressed a neuropsychological question (Pascual-Leone et al., 1994). There were some early misunderstandings of the spatial specificity of the technique, but recent, elegant work by Paus, Fox, George, Siebner, and their colleagues, among others, have laid this concern to rest. The technique needs to be used responsibly, of course, but the ongoing process of monitoring the long-term effects of TMS and new results from combining TMS and neuroimaging are proving the technique to be safe when used within certain boundaries.

Questions that come within the remit of TMS run the gamut of neuropsychological box files—perception, memory, attention, language, numeracy, priming, eye movements, action selection, plasticity, and awareness, and it is these questions our book attempts to address. Several excellent books already exist on the use of TMS in clinical neurophysiology (e.g., Mills, 1999) and neuropsychiatry (George and Belmaker, 2000), and some collected volumes provide an overview of TMS in several fields (Paulus et al., 1999; Rushworth and Walsh, 1999; Pascual-Leone et al., 2002). These volumes have allowed us to be very selective about what we chose to review, and we hope that those familiar with TMS, who might wonder at some of the omissions, will appreciate that we have tried to write a book that we believe is right for a particular area of cognitive neuropsychology at a particular point in time, rather than a book on "all there is to know about TMS" (which is, after all, more than we know). What is omitted is so because these other volumes cover those topics perfectly well, and there is really no need for another in-depth description of motor thresholds, the silent period, D and I waves, and many other aspects of TMS that, although fundamental to motor physiology, have proved, so far at least, to have limited use in cognitive neuropsychology. We do not cover other aspects in detail because they have not been applied yet to cognitive questions, although they clearly have important potential. Paired-pulse studies, for example, have not become a force in the study of TMS and cognition, though we anticipate this particular application of TMS will grow rapidly and yield hitherto unexpected findings (e.g., Oliveri et al., 2000). We could have written a chapter on phosphenes (and would have enjoyed doing so), but this topic also has been reviewed adequately elsewhere

(Marg, 1991; Marg and Rudiak, 1994), so we have limited our discussion of phosphenes to those studies that have used them to address a particular cognitive or methodological question. A similar rationale applies to our omission of studies of cortical excitability in migraineurs (Chronicle and Mulleners, 1996; Afra et al., 1998; Aurora et al., 1998) and other neurological conditions.

The use of TMS has reached maturity in clinical neurophysiology and in studies of motor functions, and it would be impossible for anyone to survey the whole field. Our hope is that the use of TMS in cognitive neuroscience will reach a similar level of maturity and that in a few years it will be all but impossible to write a short and general book on TMS and cognition such as our present effort.

ACKNOWLEDGMENTS

Many friends and colleagues provided encouragement and help as we prepared
this book and allowed us to plunder their minds for help in the things we did
not know or did not know well enough or, as we sometimes discovered, thought
we knew too well. Some read most of the manuscript, and we believe they are
making full recoveries—we wish them well; some read sections or chapters, and
others answered our questions on their area of expertise or made free with their
figures, data, or ears. It is a pleasure to name as many as we can remember:
Michael Alexander, Vahe Amassian, Anthony Barker, David Bartrés-Faz, Joaquim
Brasil-Neto, Alfonso Caramazza, Leonardo Cohen, Peter Collins, Alan Cowey,
Roger Cracco, Albert Galaburda, Massimo Gangitano, Silke Göbel, Jordan Graf-
man, Mark Hallett, Roy Hamilton, Peter Houseman, Stephen Jackson, Chi-
Hung Juan, Julian Keenan, Ray Klein, Masahito Kobayashi, Stephen Kosslyn,
Steve Lomber, Fumiko Maeda, Felix Mottaghy, Margaret O'Connor, Maximil-
iano Oliveri, Daniel Press, Edwin Robertson, John Rothwell, Michael Rutter,
Norihiro Sadato, Clif Saper, Mark Thall, Hugo Theoret, Mark Thivierge, Gregor
Thut, Robert Turner, Antoni Valero, Josep Valls-Sole, and Eric Wassermann. Our
own research and costs specifically related to our work on this book have been
funded generously, and we are grateful to the Royal Society, the McDonnell-Pew
Foundation, the Queen's College Oxford, the Dr. Hadwen Research Trust, the

Medical Research Council, the National Eye Institute, the Oxford MRC IRC, National Institute of Mental Health, the Goldberg Foundation, the Milton Fund, the National Alliance of Research in Schizophrenia and Depression, and the Stanley Vada Foundation.

Particular thanks must go to Matthew Rushworth and Lauren Stewart, who read some drafts and all of the completed manuscript, and to Amanda Ellison and José María Tormos, without whose help—no, we can't bear to think about the consequences of that.

Transcranial Magnetic Stimulation

INTRODUCTION: COGNITIVE RESOLUTION

You've never had it so good

—*U.S. political slogan 1952, reiterated by British prime minister Harold Macmillan addressing the people on the state of the economy, 1957*

There never has been a better time to be a cognitive neuroscientist. Cognitive neuroscience is defined as broadly as its parent disciplines psychology and neuroscience, and at its core stand the central questions provided by a century of psychology that have to be answered in neurological terms. These questions currently are pigeonholed within perception, attention, memory, action, imagery, language, and consciousness studies. We find ourselves at a point in history where the techniques available have advanced to meet questions that have been awaiting them—and there is a burden on us to make good this opportunity. Peter Medawar thought that it wasn't worth talking to anyone who didn't believe the discovery of the structure of DNA to be the most important discovery of the twentieth century; the same positivity currently exists in the cognitive brain sciences at the beginning of this twenty-first century. Brain-imaging methods have created a new positivism in the quest to understand the neural basis of cognition and now are being applied to the study of all cognitive functions.

The term *brain imaging* covers several techniques, the mainstays in the cognitive sciences being positron emission tomography (PET), functional magnetic resonance imaging (fMRI), magnetoencephalography (MEG), and event-related potentials (ERPs). These methods have one thing in common: they record brain activity of some sort and correlate the activity patterns with behavior. If one wants to know which human brain areas are involved in color or motion perception (Lueck et al., 1994; Zeki et al., 1993; Watson et al., 1993; Hadjikhani et al., 1998), spatial attention or eye movements (Corbetta et al., 1991, 1993, 1995; Perry and Zeki, 2000), the selection or generation of actions (Rushworth et al., 1998; Schluter et al., 1998, 1999), language processing (Price, Wise, and Frackowiack, 1996), imagining (Kosslyn et al., 1999), or even the processing of sights unseen (Barbur et al., 1993; Baseler, Morland, and Wandell, 1999), there are innumerable papers awaiting inspection (and of course demanding citation). If one wants to know something of the temporal nature of processing of different stimulus properties or response patterns, there is a plethora of ERP papers, particularly in vision (Luck and Hillyard, 1994), attention (Mangun and Hillyard, 1988), and memory (Wilding and Rugg, 1996; Allen and Rugg, 1997). And if one wishes to combine something of the temporal and spatial maps of brain functions, the "what" and "where" of these processes can be combined in MEG studies (e.g., Salmelin et al., 1994; Holliday, Anderson, and Harding, 1997) or in event-related fMRI (Buckner et al., 1996). We indeed have never had it so good because we have never had anything like it at all until now.

YOU CAN'T STUDY FUNCTION WITHOUT INTERVENTION

Brain imaging methods, for all their advantages, do not render obsolete the techniques that preceded them. Knowing which brain areas are activated preferentially during a task or when two processes diverge temporally are unlikely, alone, to provide explanations of the mechanisms by which stimuli are processed and sensory inputs result in experience and behavior. Indeed, quite the reverse is the case; brain imaging actually brings into sharp focus the need for other techniques—for example, by raising questions that can be answered only by single-unit recording or by generating hypotheses for lesion studies. Neuropsychological studies of patients had been hampered for many years by the inability to locate precisely the lesions in interesting subjects. With anatomical MRI scans, we can see patients' lesions, select patients according to the anatomical locus of damage, and thus test those patients with circumscribed lesions and subtle deficits that previously would have slipped through the net (e.g., Schoppig et al., 1999). We even can reconstruct the lesions of patients who have died (Damasio et al., 1994). Neuropsychology has been thought of as having poor spatial resolution, but it is actually *exactly* as precise as the imaging method used to produce the anatomical scan.

It is without doubt wonderful and scientifically illuminating to see snapshots of the brain in action, but to attain an understanding of the mechanisms by which the brain carries out its various functions we need to go beyond the correlations established by fMRI, PET, ERPs, and MEG and establish a chain of cause and necessity between brain activation and perceptions and action, which can be achieved only by reverse engineering the brain (Walsh, 2000), by selectively removing components from information processing, and by assessing their impact on the output. Neuropsychological studies of patients (e.g., Critchley, 1953; Milner, 1966; Shallice, 1988) and lesion studies of animals (e.g., Riopelle and Ades, 1953; Riopelle et al., 1953; Butter, 1968, 1969, 1972; Iwai and Mishkin, 1969; Cowey and Gross, 1970; Gross, Cowey, and Manning, 1971; Gross, 1978; Walsh and Butler, 1996) have been reverse engineering brains for several decades, and the first flood of imaging studies served to show just how successful these methods were. The legacy of early work with patients and monkeys has been not only to associate particular functions with regions of the brain, but also to provide the very vocabulary and grammar of our thinking on brain processes: Marr's modular view of the brain followed Warrington's demonstrations of category specific agnosias (see Marr, 1982); Zeki's physiological resurrection of sensory specialization built on case studies of color or motion deficits (see Zeki, 1993); and the notion of parallel processing came not from anatomy or computational neuroscience but from classical models of psychological information processing (see Donders, 1969; Posner, 1978; Meyer et al., 1988; Miller, 1988; Coles et al., 1995) and of neuropsychological dissociations—the list could go on (see Shallice, 1988). Psychologists also have spent the best part of a century carrying out studies in which specific stages of processing are blocked or interfered with effectively by using dual-task and masking paradigms (Pashler, 1998). These studies are not usually considered in the same light as lesion studies, but their effects and the kinds of knowledge they reveal are similar. There is no competition between the different methods available, but rather an alliance necessitated by the different shortcomings of each; indeed, all the methods available to the cognitive neuroscientist often appear inadequate in the face of some of the problems we are trying to solve.

In this book, we are concerned with a technique that emerged during the same period as neuroimaging. It is called transcranial magnetic stimulation (TMS), and it has opened a new avenue in reverse engineering the human brain's role in behavioral and cognitive functions. In TMS, a brief, intense magnetic field is applied to the scalp. This field induces electrical activity in the cortex, effectively disorganizing neural processing in that region of the cortex and thus disrupting normal functioning for a few milliseconds. This effect has been termed a *virtual lesion* (Pascual-Leone et al., 1999a; Walsh and Rushworth, 1999) and the product a *virtual patient* (Walsh and Cowey, 1998). Attempts to stimulate the brain magnetically go back more than a century, and in chapter 2 we tell the story of the remarkable struggle behind the achievement. In chapter 3, we describe some technical and ethical aspects of TMS, and in chapter 4 we give a guide to how to use the different types of TMS to ask empirical questions. The aim of chapters 3 and 4 is not to give an exhaustive "how to" guide to TMS, but to supply the prospective experimenter with a baseline of technical and practical procedural information (more detailed accounts can be found in Mills, 1999; Paulus et al., 1999; Pascual-Leone et al., 2002). The subsequent chapters bring into focus the successes (and some failures) of the technique to date and concentrate on those findings that we believe would have remained hidden without specific recourse to TMS or that highlight some particular aspect of its promise. Rather than deal with each domain of cognitive psychology (perception, attention, and so on), we have divided the chapters according to the conceptual style of the questions addressed.[1] Thus, in chapter 5, we explore the uses to which single-pulse TMS has been put in asking questions about the timing of processes, and in chapter 6 we assess the ways in which TMS—single or repetitive pulse (rTMS)—has been used to look at dynamic interactions between different cortical areas and to produce paradoxical improvements in behavior. Chapter 7 details TMS studies that have revealed changes in the roles of cortical areas as a result of development or reorganization on time scales ranging from milliseconds to years. In chapter 8, we take TMS to the neuropsychological patients, not as a therapeutic tool but as a means of using the patient as an interesting preparation—which neuropsychologists have been doing for several decades. Finally, we see how TMS already has been combined with PET and fMRI and look to the future place of TMS in the armory of cognitive neuropsychology. Before moving on, however, we need to stake out the territory of TMS: Why is it needed at all, how does it complement other techniques, and what is so important about establishing the necessity of cortical activations?

EXPERIMENTAL SPACE-TIME

"Space by itself, and time by itself, are doomed to fade away into mere shadows, and only a kind of unity between the two will preserve an independent reality."

—*Hermann Minkowski, physicist*

The strengths of fMRI, ERPs, and MEG lie in their ability to sample activity in small volumes of brain tissue (fMRI) and in small windows of time (ERPs) or to combine measurements of magnetic fields generated by brain activity into

1. We are grateful to Professor Ray Klein for suggestions on the organization of the book: our first outline was indeed divided according to sensory and motor functions.

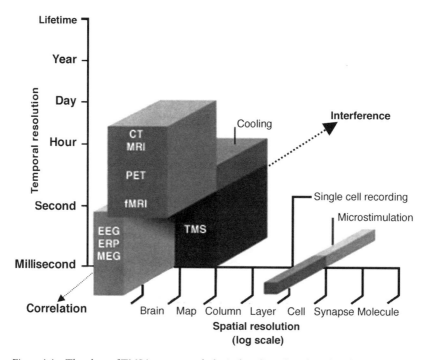

Figure 1.1 The place of TMS in neuropsychological studies is best thought of in terms of the "problem space" it occupies. This figure shows the spatial and temporal resolution of TMS compared with other techniques. However, it is not just space and time that make TMS indispensable; it is the ability of TMS transiently to interfere with functions where other techniques correlate brain activity with functions. The different volumes occupied by each of the techniques reflects the fact that when one selects a technique, one is also making a selection about the kind of question one can ask within the defined problem space. (From Walsh and Cowey, 2000, with permission.)

small segments of space and time (MEG). The relative spatial and temporal resolutions of these methods in part define the area of cognitive problem space they occupy. For TMS, the domain of most obvious interest is the temporal element it can add to the lesion paradigm. Figure 1.1 presents just one way of thinking about the consequences of spatial and temporal resolution. A simple conclusion one can draw from this figure is that ERPs cannot address questions regarding the localization of function, and fMRI can address localization but not time. Neither of these views is strictly true in any case, but the important point is that this is not the right way to think about the application of techniques and can lead to many sterile experiments (TMS ones included) in which the lack of a functional or psychological hypothesis is masked by the apparent power of the method being used. The important level of resolution is neither temporal resolution nor spatial resolution; it is *cognitive resolution*—that is, the ability of the technique to tell us something *new* about brain processes. Visual psychophysics, for example, does not have any spatial or temporal resolution in the sense that it measures or stimulates brain activity, but the insights from its functional resolution are the keystone of any experiment in visual perception. There are two main features of cognitive resolution: one is whether the technique in question establishes causal connections between a neural element and an apparently correlated behavior; the other is the range of questions that come within its remit. TMS differs from the imaging techniques in both features because it can establish the necessity of an area for a given function rather than a correlation of brain activity with behavior. TMS also differs from the other techniques in the types of questions it can tackle. This is a complex issue and recurs at several stages later in the book. Rather than go into detail, we offer a few examples here to illustrate the point. There is a longstanding debate concerning whether activity in extrastriate visual areas is sufficient for awareness of visual attributes (see Cowey and Stoerig, 1991). Patients with lesions to V1 have been studied in attempts to resolve the issue, but whenever the subjects are presented with visual stimuli, *all* remaining pathways are stimulated, leaving room for different interpretations of the results. With TMS, it is possible to stimulate extrastriate areas in isolation and show that they are necessary but not sufficient for awareness of visual attributes (Cowey and Walsh, 2000; Pascual-Leone and Walsh, 2001). In chapter 5, we also discuss an experiment by Lemon, Johansson, and Westling (1995) in which a complex motor task is analyzed on-line in a manner that would not be amenable to any other method.

Another example of the cognitive resolving power of TMS is the role it plays in demonstrating the necessity of V1 in visual imagery (Kosslyn et al.,

1999; see chapter 6). Again, the debate persisted because V1 is active whenever visual stimuli are presented, and it wasn't possible to use imaging to clarify whether this activity was meaningful or simply noise due to back projections from other areas. Results from the application of TMS over V1, however, show that this area is necessary for normal visual imagery. A final example comes from studies that began with the observation that rTMS to the right or left dorsolateral prefrontal cortex induces reductions in regional cerebral blood flow. The meaning of this change could be assessed only by applying TMS to disrupt a function associated with this area to show that the induced blood flow effects determined behavioral performance (Mottaghy et al., 2000; see chapter 8). More details of these studies and other examples of the role of TMS are contained in the relevant chapters.

REVERSIBILITY

You can't unscramble scrambled eggs.

—*American proverb*

The traditions to which cognitive studies using TMS belong are those of neuropsychology and experimental psychology. The logic of lesion analysis employed in most TMS studies is the same as that used in neuropsychology, but there are important differences that allow TMS to go beyond the findings from patients and systematically to pursue effects that it would not be possible to investigate in patients. With patients, one is presented with the problem of making inferences about normal brain function on the basis of experiments with an abnormal preparation. The longer the lesion has been in place, the less one can be confident about the extent to which compensatory plasticity has caused areas to change functions or tasks to be performed in different ways. Using TMS as a reversible lesion technique means that normal subjects can be studied, and because the effects of TMS last only a few tens of milliseconds, the problem of reorganization is bypassed. The reversibility of virtual lesions also means that individual subjects can be used as their own controls and in studies of learning and transfer at different stages of skill acquisition. Some of the advantages of reversible lesions are already well known from the animal literature, and pharmacological studies in humans also have been used inventively (cf., Lomber, 1999; Malpeli, 1999; Martin and Chez, 1999).

Lomber (1999), whose own work relies on reversible lesions induced by cooling the cortex, provides an insightful and detailed rationale for using reversible deactivation techniques rather than classical lesion methods, and much of his commentary applies to TMS; indeed, TMS studies have much to learn from the literature on reversible lesions induced by cooling or pharmacological manipulations (e.g., Martin-Elkins, George, and Horel, 1989; Horel, 1996; Hupe et al., 1999a,b, 2001; Lomber, 1999; Lomber, Payne, and Horel, 1999; Payne and Lomber, 1999). The generic advantage of reversibly disrupting a region of the brain is that it allows one to overcome what Lomber (1999) calls "the specter of neural compensations," the ability of other brain areas to take over the function being investigated. If one removes a brain area or examines a patient who has suffered permanent brain damage, then one is studying the function of the tissue that remains as much as the tissue that has been removed (see chapter 8 for further discussion). Removal of a brain area also incurs damage to distal sites caused by severed vessels, ablated white matter, and degenerated neurons along the tracts serving the removed area. One only can suspect that the technical competence and hypothesis-driven approach demanded by cooling techniques has prevented their being in more widespread use, but the ability to control the duration of inactivation, the short recovery time, and the small areas of tissue to which cooling can be limited (between 2 and 100 mm^3 depending on the type of probe used) may encourage more labs to adopt the reversible-lesion approach in animals and to generate experiments on cortical regions that cannot be accessed by TMS in human subjects (see chapters 3 and 4).

Throughout the book, we have selected experiments to illustrate what TMS can contribute to cognitive neuroscience: those contributions may be to confirm the findings of other studies or to refute them; to replicate patients or to go beyond the findings from them; to address problems that cannot be approached by other techniques or to find new problems. The new problems herald a new era in cognitive neuroscience—TMS has arrived, with many questions in brain and behavior awaiting it.

MAGNETS AND MINDS IN HISTORY

We have little idea at present of the importance they may have ten or twenty years hence.

—*Michael Faraday in a letter to Hans Christian Oersted concerning scientific discoveries, 1850*

In science, theories and the experiments used to substantiate them often are driven by the development of new methodologies. The creation of new tools and techniques has a dramatic impact on the kinds of discoveries and insights that subsequently emerge. The fact that theories often are yoked to the development of new technologies is particularly apparent in the neurosciences. Camillo Golgi (1843–1926), influenced by his friend Giulio Bizzozero and Rudolf Virchow's book *Zellularpathologie,* decided to devote himself to the study of the structure of the nervous system. Golgi had to overcome his father's advice, a family physician in the small town of Corteno (Lombardy, Italy), that he ought to try to make a livelihood and forget senseless pastimes. Indeed, financial needs eventually forced Golgi to become the resident physician in the Ospizio-Cronici in Abbiategrasso, but the seeds of scientific inquiry were already deeply rooted in his soul. Golgi worked at night by candlelight in a crude laboratory set up in the kitchen of his home and here, almost serendipitously, he discovered a technique for staining the arborization of individual neurons, the "*reazione nera*" (silver-chromate staining method). Golgi's staining method permitted Santiago Ramón y Cajal (1852–1934) to formulate the neuronal theory that opposed the view of a reticular nervous system held by many at the time, including Golgi himself. Cajal, too, was born in a small village, Petilla de Aragón (Spain), also the son of a country doctor. As in Golgi's case, Cajal's father feared that his son would never earn enough to sustain a living. Cajal was artistically inclined and showed an interest in drawing while otherwise being declared lazy and dull by teachers and summer job employers. Drawings of bones of the animals his father hunted kindled Cajal's interest in anatomy and led to his study of medicine. His careful drawings of what he saw under the microscope eventually were to become the sure demonstration of the neuron theory, in addition to being works of art in their own right. Cajal had seen examples of Golgi's staining method in 1887 while he served as judge in an examination for a professorship at the University of Madrid and quickly had started experimenting with modifications of the staining method. Therefore, it was in using Golgi's method that Cajal made most of his seminal discoveries, a fact he readily and frequently acknowledged. Nevertheless, the tension between these two giants of modern neuroscience (figure 2.1) carried all the way to their acceptance speeches for their shared Noble Prize in Medicine in 1906. Golgi aggressively attacked Cajal and defended the reticular hypothesis of brain structure, and the latter gave a clear exposition of facts, including the demonstration that Golgi's own preparations actually showed free nerve endings, overlapping nerve fibers, and individual nerve cells. Cajal concluded: "it is the sad truth that almost nobody can completely free oneself from the tradition and spirit of his times, not even the wise man of Padua." The fact is that Golgi's staining method made Cajal's conceptual revolution possible by providing a means of experimentally testing a theory: Cajal needed to be able to see what he looked at, but the ability to look required the appropriate instruments and the preexisting concept of what to look for.

There are many other examples of the interaction between new technological developments and novel theories in neuroscience. Hodgkin and Huxley's (1939)

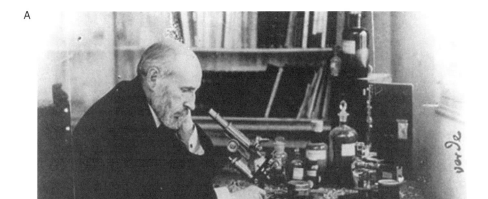

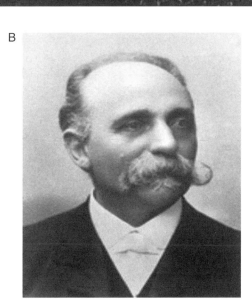

Figure 2.1 (*a*) Santiago Ramón y Cajal is depicted in a photograph taken by himself, a very accomplished hobby photographer, in his study while he was living in the Calle Pizarro, in Valencia, Spain. (*b*) Camillo Golgi.

elucidation of the properties of the action potential allowed intimate knowledge of the electrophysiology underlying neuronal interactions, and it has shaped our thinking about the way in which neurons work and respond to inputs. More recently, technical advances in engineering have led to novel neuroimaging tools that have vastly enriched our understanding of the relationship between structure and function in the central nervous system and have given rise to scientific inquiries in topics ranging from cerebrovascular pathology to theories of consciousness. Over the course of a few years, discoveries such as these have revolutionized the neurosciences and given rise to myriad theories that could be formulated only because of the new methods to generate them in the first place.

Similarly, the rich and colorful history of magnetic brain stimulation, at all stages in its development, illustrates the ways in which technical advances influence the scope of scientific inquiry. TMS is the product of a revolution in science that is more than 150 years in the making. The history begins with Michael Faraday's crucial discovery of electromagnetic induction, continues through the turn of the century with devices used to induce visual percepts, and eventually culminates in Anthony Barker's recent development of TMS. Now that TMS exists as a technique in its own right, it promises to set the stage for the next generation of discoveries and theories about the structure and function of sensory and cognitive processes. However, this shall be the case only if carefully constructed rational models are developed that can then make use of TMS to put them to test. In Thomas Kuhn's words, "consciously or not, the decision to employ a particular piece of apparatus and to use it in a particular way carries an assumption that only certain situations will arise. There are instrumental as well as theoretical expectations, and they play a decisive role in scientific development" (1970).

MAGNETIC PERSONALITIES: ANCIENT ROOTS OF MAGNETISM

According to one legend, the first discovery of a magnetic substance in the Western world was by the shepherd Magnus in 1000 B.C. Magnus was walking on the trails of Mysia and noted that his feet were drawn to the ground by the tacks in his sandals. He must have had an inquisitive mind because legend tells us that he dug in the earth and uncovered the cause of the phenomenon: a stone that he called "magnetite"—a magnetic oxide of iron (Fe_3O_4), which later came to be known as lodestone (Gilbert, 1600; Marg, 1991). Other historical accounts indicate that the term *magnetism* comes not from this lone shepherd, but from the Magnetes, the people of ancient Magnesia in Thessaly, where such lodestones were found.

In the Middle Ages, under the influence of superstition, magnets were attributed great and bizarre medicinal powers (indeed, they still are so attributed today; surf the Web and you shall find magnetic "cures" for everything from headaches to hemorrhoids). Magnets were thought to relieve arthritis and gout, draw poison from wounds, reverse baldness, and cure epilepsy. In the sixteenth century, the physician and alchemist Theophrastus Paracelsus (1493–1541) claimed that all persons possessed magnetic powers, and it was under the influence of this theory that two centuries later the Viennese physician Franz Anton Mesmer (1734–1815) named these alleged innate forces *animal magnetism*. The end of the eighteenth and beginning of the nineteenth centuries saw "mesmerism" or "magnetism" become increasingly widespread throughout Europe and the United States (Gauld, 1992). Remarkable cases of "miracle cures" made Mesmer both a sought-after healer and a most controversial figure in Vienna and later in Paris. A notable example is the case of Miss Paradis, a young pianist blind since the age of four to whom Mesmer restored partial vision by "magnetizing" her. The patient and her family initially were delighted with the "cure," but when they questioned Mesmer and magnetism Mesmer and his followers threatened them aggressively and bitterly. Mesmer was not to be ignored. He was a flamboyant and obstinate individual who held his ideas with unshakable conviction, gaining large numbers of followers and faithful believers. Essentially following Paracelsus, he believed that all living bodies contained "magnetic fluid" that generated "tides" that, if disorganized, resulted in any number of pathologies such as convulsive and fainting fits, hysteria, ophthalmoplegia, delirium, aches and pains. Through "animal magnetism," it was possible for properly trained and gifted individuals (such as Mesmer himself) to revive the impaired tides of a patient's own magnetic fluid, hence restoring the nervous system to "harmony." The use of magnets, Mesmer concluded, was not necessary; simply the "passing" of the hands over the patient's body would funnel the animal magnetism and exert the curative effect. In 1789, Eberhard Gmelin published the first reference to "mesmeric anesthesia." Jules Cloquet is often credited with the first major surgery performed in 1829 using "mesmeric sleep" as the sole form of anesthesia. In 1842, W. Squire Ward amputated the gangrenous left leg of James Wombell, who had been put into "mesmeric sleep" by William Topham. Phrenology and mesmerism notably combined into "phrenomagnetism" and were quickly popularized by such journals as *The Phreno-Magnet*, which Spencer T. Hall started in Sheffield in 1843. The notion of "focal" applications of animal magnetism over phrenologically identified "organs" of the brain and cognition in order to modify patient's alignments, to "enhance morality and human welfare," to "re-educate instead of punishing," and to "reveal the full expression of individuals' potentialities" captured the imagination of many. The notions are remarkably resonant of José María Delgado's concept of a "psychocivilized society" to be achieved by modulation of activity in focal brain structures through the use of implanted depth electrodes (Delgado, 1965, 1980). The fact that Spencer Hall started his society in Sheffield had no influence, as far as we are aware, on Anthony Barker's subsequent development of the modern magnetic stimulators at the University of Sheffield in the 1980s.

Fortunately, the principles of magnetism upon which TMS relies borrow little from these early applications of magnets, animal magnetism, and phrenomagnetism. Instead, magnetic brain stimulation is grounded in the physical sciences and has its origins in the elegant discoveries of one of the pioneers of electromagnetism, Michael Faraday (1791–1867). Nevertheless, the popular belief in the power of magnetism has continued through the ages. Exposure to small-intensity magnetic fields reportedly can speed up bone formation and fracture healing, control chronic pain, and reduce inflammation. The sale of magnets for the treatment of a long list of ailments has become a multi-million-dollar industry. "Hand passing" as a method of healing is still popular and is discussed frequently not only in the tabloid press but also in pseudoscientific publications and on television science programs. In the past few years, a rapidly growing number of putative therapeutic applications of TMS are being claimed for such disparate conditions as depression, schizophrenia, obsessive-compulsive disorders, Parkinson's disease, posttraumatic stress disorder, epilepsy, tics, dystonia, or myoclonus (see chapter 8). The link between mesmerism and modern magnetic stimulation lies only in the irrationality of some of the beliefs that accompany them. The important difference between the modern age of TMS and the "New Age" of magnetic therapies is that the applications of TMS are based on physics and physiology.

Famous Coils

On 29 August 1831, the British chemist, physicist, and natural philosopher Michael Faraday (figure 2.2) realized that he had discovered something remarkable—something he believed "may probably have great influence in some of the most important effects of electric currents." Faraday was one of ten children of a blacksmith and had had little formal education until 1813, when at the age of twenty-two, he became Sir Humphry Davy's (1778–1829) assistant at the Royal Institution. Davy, the discoverer of the respiratory effects of "laughing gas" (nitrous oxide) and the inventor of the "safety lamp" for use in mines where methane was present, hence preventing explosions, was a meticulous man. His assistant, Faraday, also kept detailed records of his countless studies in laboratory notebooks. On that particular day, 29 August 1831, based on what he had observed, Faraday began a new counting scheme for the experiments in his notebook, beginning over again at number one. The experiment he then proceeded to describe is that in which he first discovered magnetic induction.

At the time of this discovery, it was already known from Luigi Galvani's (1737–1798) experiments that nervous tissue had *something* to do with electricity. Galvani had found that frogs' legs twitch when the muscles are placed against two different metal conductors. He concluded that these findings proved that frog legs and indeed all muscles have internal electricity. The fascinating debate

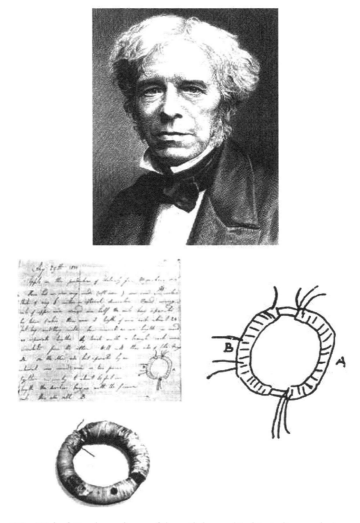

Figure 2.2 Michael Faraday and one of the coils he used in his studies on electromagnetic induction. Illustration of the first magnetic induction coil, sketched by Faraday in his laboratory notebook on 29 August, 1831, and an inset from the notebook.

between Alessandro Volta (1745–1827) and Galvani was ongoing. Volta believed that the frog leg and indeed any muscle simply provided the "salt solution" for the electricity to flow between two electrodes. Both Volta and Galvani turned out to be somewhat right. Certainly only some tissues, as countless ensuing experiments came to demonstrate, can be induced to contract or change by the passing of current. Belief in the power of electricity grew, and in 1755 the French physician Charles Le Roy generated electrophosphenes in an attempt to cure a blind twenty-one-year-old Englishman called Granger. Le Roy wound conducting wires around Granger's head and led one wire to his leg. The array was connected to a charged Leyden jar, and twelve shocks were administered in the hope (faint in Le Roy's view) that sight would be restored (figure 2.3). Along with the pain of the stimulation, the patient did perceive vivid phosphenes and underwent the treatment several times in the following days. He remained blind. In the context of such experiments, in 1757 the Italian naturalist Felice Gaspar Fontana (1730–1805; figure 2.4) and Leopoldo Caldani (1725–1813) applied electric stimulation to the cerebral cortex of decapitated criminals and to muscles of cadaver limbs. The results of these experiments were reportedly so fantastic and frightening for the time that in Prussia experiments on beheaded corpses became outlawed in 1804. Caldani and Fontana went on to conduct experiments on a conscious man during trephination, unequivocal forerunners of the experiments with direct electric stimulation of the cortex to become widespread in the following century. In 1838, Carlo Matteucci (1811–68) introduced the term *muscle current* to describe the activity of muscle tissue previously referred to as "animal electricity." Ten years later Emil Du Bois–Reymond (1818–96) demonstrated a direct relationship between electric current and nerve cell activity, and G-B. Guillaume Duchenne de Boulogne (1806–75) became the first to use electricity in the study of disease, both for diagnostic as well as therapeutic goals (faradization). In *L'électrisation localisée* (1855), Duchenne describes the method founded in the observation that a current from two electrodes applied to the wet skin can stimulate muscles without damaging the skin. In 1872, in the third edition of *L'électrisation localisée,* Duchenne included a chapter he titled "The Mechanism of Expression" (first published in

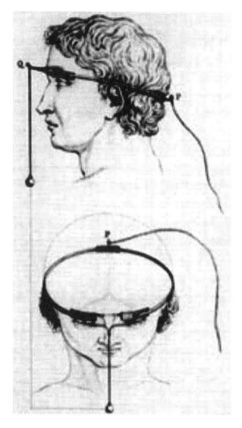

Figure 2.3   Charles Le Roy stimulated a blind patient through the retina (Q) and cortex (P) in 1755. The electrodes were connected to a Leyden jar, which discharged shocks to the patient. The patient reported vivid phosphenes but remained blind.

1862). Figure 2.5 shows Duchenne pointing out that "the method of electrisation" allows the study of the function of facial muscles and their contribution to emotional expression. Among other applications of faradization, Duchenne describes the case of a woman admitted to the Charité, "whither she had been brought the night before stifled by carbonic oxide." Duchenne "very soon brought back the pulse and breathing, and caused the coma to disappear" by ap-

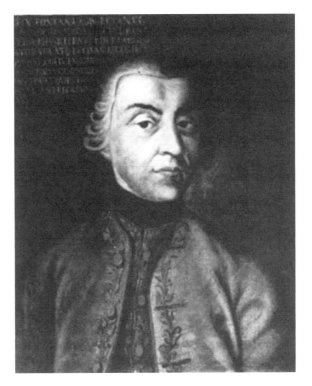

Figure 2.4 Felice Gaspar Fontana, who contributed to anatomical, pharmacological, and electrical stimulation studies of nervous tissue.

plying "faradization of the skin of the praecordia." In the wake of such findings, it is not surprising that Giovanni Aldini (1762–1834; figure 2.6), Galvani's nephew, experimented with electric "therapy" to treat psychoses and melancholia and even to revive the dead ("Essai theorique et experimental sur le galvanisms," 1804). Certainly here lie the origins of electroshock and cardioversion. Transcranial magnetic stimulation cannot revive the dead, but it may work for some academic careers.

In his seminal experiment, Faraday wound two pieces of wire on opposite sides of an iron ring. He observed the disturbance of a magnetic needle placed

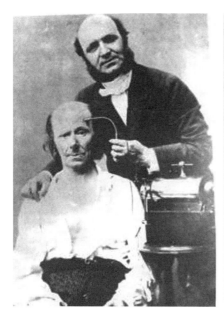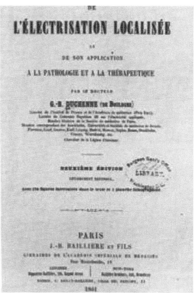

Figure 2.5   G-B. Duchenne de Boulogne demonstrating contraction of the frontalis muscle caused by faradic stimulation and the title page of Duchenne's work on electrotherapy.

near one wire coil (coil B) when an electric current was connected or disconnected to the other coil (coil A). This simple observation demonstrated that an electric current had been induced in B by passing a current through A. Later Faraday showed that the iron ring, which enhanced the induction of current in coil B by "guiding" the magnetic field between the two coils, was nonessential and that "action at a distance" could be reproduced with two closely positioned air-cored coils.

Despite the significance of his findings, Faraday described his work with modesty and skepticism, stating "I am busy just now again on electro-magnetism, and I think I have got hold of a good thing, but I can't say. It may be a weed instead of a fish that, after all my labor, I may at last pull up" (qtd. in James, 1993). It was no weed; it was Faraday's discovery of magnetic induction, which laid the foundations that during the nineteenth century allowed electricity to be turned

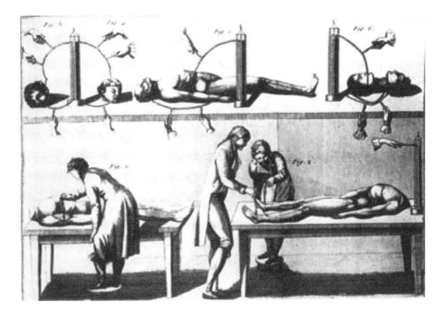

Figure 2.6 Copper plate from Giovanni Aldini (1804) showing electrical stimulation experiments performed on human bodies following decapitation.

from a scientific curiosity into a powerful technology. It was also this discovery, more than any other, that established the first principles from which all subsequent studies on the neurophysiological effects of magnetic stimulation have been derived.

In the years following Faraday's discovery, numerous investigators attempted in vain to induce physiological effects using magnetic fields. Lord Kelvin (1824–1907), for example, cites one example of an enormous, yet ineffective, electromagnet constructed by Lord Lindsay, which was "so large that it would admit between its poles the head of any person who wished to test whether a strong magnetic field would have any sensible effect" (Thompson, 1910). What these early would-be neurophysiologists overlooked was a simple principle that Faraday had realized when he originally discovered induction. In a sealed letter penned in 1832 to John George Childer, the secretary for the Royal

Society, Faraday had written: "Certain of the results of the investigations . . . lead me to believe that magnetic action is progressive and requires time; i.e. that when a magnet acts upon a distant magnet or piece of iron, the influencing cause (which I may call for the moment magnetism) proceeds gradually from the magnetic bodies, and requires time for transition. . . . I think also, that I see reason for supposing that electric induction (of tension) is also performed in a similar progressive way" (qtd. in James, 1993).

Indeed, the critical variable for magnetic induction is not the strength of the electromagnet used but rather the rate of change of magnetic field strength over time. It is the flux of the magnetic field that induces current in a system, whether that system is a copper wire or a network of neurons. Thus, it was not until the development of alternating magnetic fields that the physiologic effects of magnetic stimulation could be observed fully.

"IT'S A PATIENT!"

On the tail of Fontana and Caldani's 1757 experiment on a conscious man during trephination, it is not surprising that direct electric stimulation of the cortex became an increasingly popular method to inquire about localized function of the brain. Even earlier, Luigi Rolando (1773–1831), after whom the central (Rolandic) sulcus is named, describes similar experiments in the classic opus *Saggio sopra la vera struttura del cervello dell' uomo e degl' animali e sopra la funzioni del sistema nervoso* (1809), which he himself engraved, printed, and bound. Rolando inserted a voltaic pile into the cerebral hemisphere of a pig and evoked violent responses of the muscles of the extremities, reaching the conclusion that the cerebral hemispheres contained a group of fibers for voluntary movement control. The massive amount of current generated by the voltaic pile presumably prevented Rolando from discovering the crossed corticopyramidal projections. Pierre Fluorens's (1794–1867) experiments on dogs and pigeons put into question the notions of localization of function in the cerebral cortex ("My experiments establish that the hemispheres of the brain do not produce any movement,") but eventually Hughlings Jackson's (1835–1911) studies of epilepsy and Gustav Fritsch

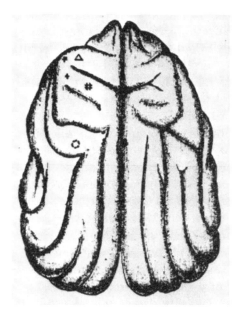

Figure 2.7   Dorsal view of a dog's brain from which Fritsch and Hitzig evoked movement by electrical stimulation. The triangle, plus sign, hash, and circle show respectively the regions from which movements of the neck, forelimb, hindlimb, and face could be elicited.

(1838–1927) and Edvard Hitzig's (1838–1907) experiments were to disprove Flu-orens's thesis, reaffirm localizationist notions of brain function, and establish corti-cal stimulation as a useful neurophysiologic method (figure 2.7).

Fritsch and Hitzig worked at Hitzig's home in Berlin and systematically explored the entire convexity of the cerebral hemisphere using platinum elec-trodes stuck through a cork and currents just strong enough "to be felt on the tongue." They demonstrated that with "electrical stimulation of the motor part one gets combined muscle contractions of the opposite part of the body." Sir David Ferrier (1843–1928) confirmed and elaborated Hitzig and Fritsch's work. Ferrier used minimal currents and electrodes placed a millimeter apart to demonstrate that he could produce isolated twitches of an eyelid, slight elevation of the angle of the mouth, or the clutching of a paw. Ferrier mapped the entire

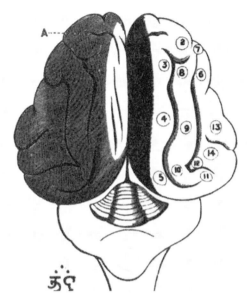

Figure 2.8   Dorsal view of a cat's brain showing where Ferrier's electrical stimulation could elicit specific responses.

cortex in meticulous experiments in different animals and finally in monkeys and realized that "there is no reason to suppose that one part of the brain is excitable and another not. The question is how the stimulation manifests itself" (figure 2.8). Ferrier demonstrated his monkeys at the 1881 International Medical Congress in London. One of the animals, made hemiplegic by motor cortex stimulation and ablation, prompted Jean-Martin Charcot (1825–93) to exclaim: "It's a patient!" Indeed, Ferrier's classic books *The Functions of the Brain* (1876) and *The Croonian Lectures on Cerebral Localization* (1890) included descriptions of Hughlings Jackson's patients and was hence among the first to link experimental animal work to clinical observations.

Many neurologists, neurosurgeons, and neurophysiologists used electric stimulation of the cortex in the following decades to make fundamental discoveries on brain organization and function. Notable achievements include

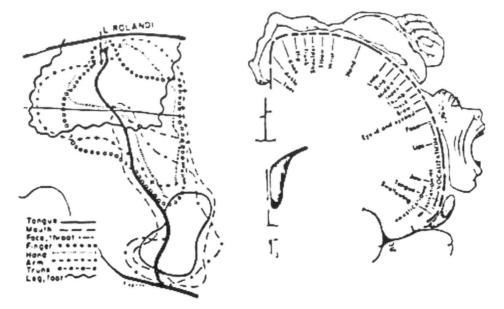

Figure 2.9 Homunculus of the motor cortical representation in the adult human as generated by Wilder Penfield and Herbert Jasper in the attempt to provide a simplified, cartoonlike summary of their findings.

Sir Victor Horsley's (1857–1916) demonstration that the effects of stimulation are modified by the brain's own generated electric currents and Charles Francois-Franck's (1849–1921) description of autonomic effects of brain stimulation. Ivan Sechenov (1829–1905) and Ivan Pavlov (1949–36) further described autonomic and reflex activity, and Rudolf Magnus (1873–1927) worked on the effects of cortical stimulation on body posture. Many other important contributions could be named for a line of investigation that culminated with Sir Charles Scott Sherrington's (1856–1952) *The Integrative Action of the Nervous System* and was applied systematically to the human brain and popularized by Wilder Penfield, Herbert Jasper, and many others (figure 2.9). Working on conscious humans during neurosurgical procedures, Penfield and coworkers (Penfield and Boldrey, 1937; Penfield and Rasmussen, 1949) recorded the cognitive effects of stimulation in different parts of the brain: experiences of the patient's past, involuntary laughter and crying, anxiety, relaxation, pleasure, dysaesthesias, pain, visual and auditory hallucinations, word-finding difficulties, agrammatisms, and vocalizations. For example, stimulation of the occipital cortex generated the patient's experience of brief flashes of light, phosphenes, as Arsène d'Arsonval had reported several years previously with use of magnetic stimulation.

VISIONARIES AND MAGNET-INDUCED VISIONS

In 1896, as a by-product of his research on the measurement of alternating current, the French physician Arsène d'Arsonval first reported the induction of phosphenes by magnetic fields (figure 2.10). In a paper entitled "Apparatus for Measuring Alternating Currents of All Frequencies," d'Arsonval wrote that "an alternating magnetic field with an intensity of 110 volts, 30 amperes and a frequency of 42 cycles per second, gives rise to, when one places the head into the coil, phosphenes and vertigo, and in some persons, syncope." D'Arsonval himself is better remembered as one of the developers of the galvanometer in 1882, and he used this device to measure the currents generated in this ground-breaking magnetic stimulation experiment (Geddes, 1991).

Perhaps because it was published in French, d'Arsonval's paper was not read by many of his contemporaries. In Vienna in 1902, Berthold Beer, who reportedly was unaware of d'Arsonval's earlier findings, conducted a survey of the research on the physiologic effects of magnetic stimulation and found that a Swiss electrical engineer by the name of E. K. Müller had, at the turn of the century, reported seeing a "flimmer" (flicker) when he applied an electromagnet to the eye (Beer, 1902). Using the very same magnet that Müller had used, Beer was able to reproduce these sensations at the edge of the visual field by placing the heads of volunteers within the coil, which was then supplied with alternating current of 15 to 20 amps (figure 2.11).

In the early twentieth century, as alternating current began to replace direct current as a source of electrical energy, it became easier for experimentalists to generate alternating magnetic fields, and with this ability the topic of "magnetophosphenes" became an increasingly popular research area. Silvanus Phillips

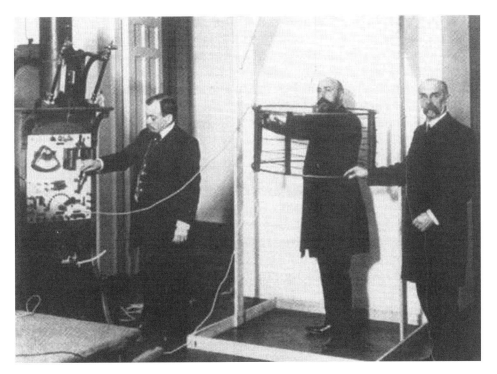

Figure 2.10 In this 1911 photograph, Arsène d'Arsonval (on the right) and two of his assistants are shown demonstrating the effects of the flow of alternating current sixteen years after d'Arsonval reported the first magnetophosphenes. Original image from the Archives of the Acadèmie de Sciences, Paris. (Reproduced from Marg, 1991.)

Thompson (figure 2.12)—who was then the renowned head of the British Institute of Electrical Engineers, the first president of the Roentgen Society, and head of the Physical Society—was attracted to the study of magnetically induced visual sensations by the anecdotal accounts of workmen in powerhouses who would experience visual phenomena when they were close to the electromagnetic coils used to dampen currents supplied to electric furnaces (Thompson, 1910). Thompson had achieved distinction in many fields as a teacher, historian, scientist and biographer: He worked on X rays, radioactivity,

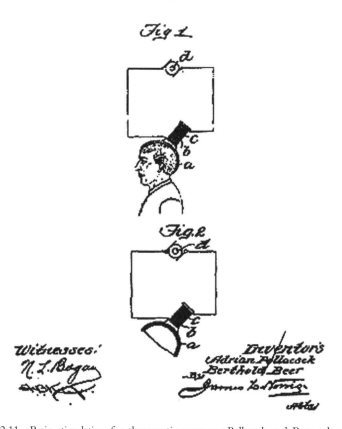

Figure 2.11 Brain stimulation for therapeutic purposes: Pollacsek and Beer submitted a patent for this device in 1902.

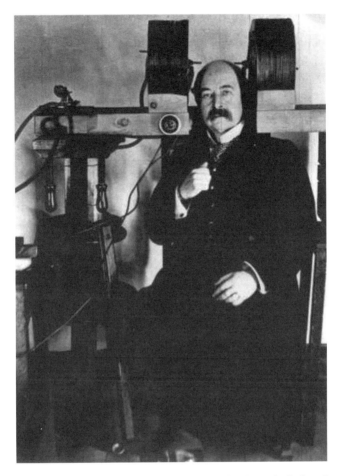

Figure 2.12   Silvanus Phillips Thompson depicted with the device he had used to induce magnetophosphenes in himself. Original image from the Archives, Imperial College, London. (Reproduced from Marg, 1991.)

telephone transmission, and color vision; he translated William Gilbert's *De magnete;* he published a biography of Lord Kelvin; and he produced influential textbooks an electromagnetism and calculus (see Lynch, 1989). With all these interests and commitments, it is perhaps understandable that Thompson was unaware of d'Arsonval's earlier work with magnetic stimulation when he constructed a large 32-turn coil (9 in. diameter and 8 in. long) in 1910 and applied up to 180 amps of power-line current to it, generating a peak maximum intensity at the center of the coil of approximately 1,400 CGS (centimeter-gram-second units, a unit that later was named after Carl Friedrich Gauss). Thompson stated that "on inserting the head into the interior of the coil, in the dark, or with the eyes closed, there is perceived over the whole region of vision a faint flickering illumination, colourless or of a slightly bluish tint" (1910). These *magnetophosphenes* (a term coined by Thompson) could be perceived with the eyes open and in the daylight. Several of his subjects also noticed a strange taste after two to three minutes of exposure to Thompson's apparatus, a perception currently inducible by TMS and probably related to transcranial activation of the facial nerve and the corda tympani.

Despite these seemingly robust findings, Knight Dunlap at Johns Hopkins University remained skeptical of the validity of Thompson's experiment (Dunlap, 1911). He believed that the loud hum produced by the current flowing through the transformer that powered the head coil had a psychological effect on subjects. In 1911, in an attempt to design a cleaner experiment, Dunlap constructed a 27-turn elliptical coil (8 in. high and 10.5 in. in diameter), which was suspended from the ceiling and could be lowered over the subject's head. To control for the possible psychological effects of suggestive sounds, subjects wore earplugs. Furthermore, when current was not flowing through the head coil, it was delivered to a resistor that caused the transformer to produce the same sound as when the current flowed through the head coil. When Dunlap tested with 200 amps of current at 60 Hz, some subjects experienced flickering phosphenes, but others did not. Looking to achieve more consistent results, Dunlap took his apparatus to a power-testing plant, where he eventually was able to increase the stimulation to 480 amps of 25 Hz current. At that point, all subjects responded, and some reported that the whole visual field was illuminated. Dunlap attributed the visual sensations produced by stimulation to "the inhibition or reinforcement of some visual excitation going on in the nerve at the time of stimulation by the magnetic field" (1911). However, he recognized that "whether currents induced in the optic pathway excite the occipital cortex directly or excite the retina primarily, is yet a matter of conjecture."

In 1911, Magnusson and Stevens constructed two coils with elliptical cross sections. These coils could be used singly or arranged coaxially, and direct or alternating current was passed through the coils surrounding subjects' heads (figure 2.13). No sensation was perceived when the direct current was flowing, but sensations were experienced when the direct-current flow was being initiated or arrested. When the direct current was initiated, subjects perceived a luminous horizontal bar moving downward. When the direct current was arrested, the luminous bar moved upward. With alternating current applied to the air-wound, head-encircling coil, flickering lights appeared and were brightest at a current frequency of 20–30 Hz. Magnusson and Stevens tried to determine at what point in the visual pathway magnetic stimulation was inducing its physiologic effects. They pursued this question by attempting to stimulate nerves outside the confines of the visual system to determine whether these nerves could be affected or if responsiveness to magnetic stimulation was a property of the retina. They carried out an unsuccessful experiment with a special coil that applied a 60 Hz alternating current to the exposed sciatic nerve of a cat. "It was hoped to determine by this [cat] experiment whether the locus of excitation in the production of visual sensations was in the sensory elements of the retina itself or in the fibers of the optic nerve. The observations must be extended before definite conclusions can be made" (Magnusson and Stevens, 1914).

More than three decades passed before more progress was made in the field of magnetic stimulation. By this time, it was known that visual sensations could be produced by stimulation of the retina, optic nerve, and occipital cortex (Geddes, 1991). In 1946, Walsh reported the induction of phosphenes using an iron-core coil placed adjacent to the eye and energized with an alternating current varying from 5 to 90 Hz. With constant alternating current in the coil, the

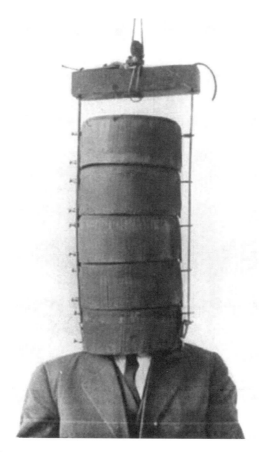

Figure 2.13   The magnetic coils used by Magnusson and Stevens. Additional sections of coils could be energized to increase the magnetic field. (Reproduced from Marg, 1991.)

visual sensation vanished in a few seconds and more rapidly when the frequency was high and the intensity low. The visual sensation could be prolonged by the subject's moving his or her eyes. Recovery usually occurred in less than a minute, and pressure to the eyes abolished the visual response. Walsh's findings were extended by Barlow and colleagues (1947), who constructed a small coil surrounding a laminated iron core. The coil was placed adjacent to one temple but not in contact with the skin. Alternating current of 10 to 40 Hz was applied, producing both colorless and colored flickering-light sensations. When the coil current was increased, the flickering light occupied more of the visual field. As in Walsh's studies, Barlow found that eye movements prolonged the effect. He also found that no phosphenes were perceived when the coil was placed over the occiput. On the basis of this evidence, he concluded that magnetophosphenes were generated through stimulation of the retina and not in the visual pathways or the visual cortex, stating that "otherwise, we cannot explain the effects of localized magnetic stimulus, pressure on the eyeball and movements of the eyeball, all of which profoundly affect phosphenes" (Barlow et al., 1947). Several other investigators went on further to characterize the nature of magnetophosphenes (Valentinuzzi, 1962; Seidel, 1968; Oster, 1970), including Lovsund et al. (1980), who performed a quantitative analysis of threshold values for the generation of magnetophosphenes and also confirmed Barlow and colleagues' earlier claims that these sensations originated in the retina.

In 1959, in order to demonstrate that an alternating magnetic field could stimulate nerves in addition to the retina, Alexander Kolin and colleagues, working in the Department of Biophysics at the University of California in Los Angeles, constructed an excitation coil surrounding a bar electromagnet with a pyramidal pole tip. Using 60 and 1,000 Hz alternating current, they found that flickering-light sensations were strongest when the pole tip was held against the occipital area or against the temple. They then demonstrated, for the first time, that an alternating magnetic field could stimulate nervous tissue in vitro. They isolated a frog sciatic-nerve-gastrocnemius-muscle preparation and looped the sciatic nerve around the pole of the magnet. Intense contraction of the gastrocnemius muscle was obtained when both 60 and 1,000 Hz were applied to the coil. To complete their investigation, they placed the nerve-muscle preparation in a Petri dish filled with saline. They placed the dish on the pole face of the magnet and applied alternating current to the coil, which resulted in tetanic contraction of the gastrocnemius muscle. This experiment offered definitive proof that a magnetic field could induce enough current to stimulate a motor nerve.

PULSED MAGNETIC FIELDS AND THE MODERN ERA
OF MAGNETIC STIMULATION

In 1965, Bickford and Fremming first used a pulsed magnetic field to twitch skeletal muscle in intact frogs, rabbits, and humans. Their system produced pulses of 2 to 3 Tesla with a 300 μs duration powered by a bank of capacitors. In six human subjects, twitches were obtained in the muscles innervating the ulnar, sciatic, and peroneal nerves. Bickford and Freeming asserted that their findings were "consistent with the hypothesis that stimulation results from eddy currents induced in the vicinity of motor neurons" (1965). Prior to this work, sinusoidal alternating current had been the primary means for powering excitation coils. High currents had been used to achieve magnetic fields of adequate strength, and the prolonged flow caused the excitation coil to become hot. Furthermore, alternating current produced a tetanic contraction when a motor nerve was stimulated by the magnetic field. However, the pulsed magnetic field produced by discharging a capacitor bank into the excitation coil typically produced a single, short-duration, biphasic (or polyphasic) damped induced-current waveform, resulting in a single twitch when a motor nerve was stimulated (Geddes, 1991).

A decade later, Anthony Barker (figure 2.14) and coworkers at the University of Sheffield were investigating the possibility of achieving velocity-selective nerve stimulation, which led them to study independently the possibility of using magnetic stimulation for clinical purposes (Barker, 1976). It soon became apparent that the technical problems of generating the large-peak magnetic field strengths and rates of change of magnetic field necessary to cause stimulation were considerable and that little was known about the required fields. Work was then initiated jointly in the Departments of Medical Physics and Clinical Engineering at the University of Sheffield to examine the technique in detail. This effort led, in 1981, to the first stimulation of the superficial peripheral nerves using a short-duration single pulse of magnetic field with the action potentials being recorded from nearby muscles (Polson, Barker, and Freeston, 1982). First, the path of the median nerve was marked out on the surface of the arm. Recording electrodes were then placed on the thenar

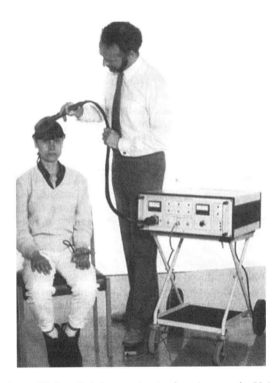

Figure 2.14 The world's first clinical magnetic stimulator in use at the University of
Sheffield in 1985, England. (Reproduced from Barker, 1991.)

eminence and connected to an electromyographic (EMG) recorder. The edge of
the excitation coil was placed on the skin over the nerve and a pulse of current
was delivered, producing a peak magnetic field of 2.2 Tesla. The thumb muscles
twitched, and an EMG response was recorded. For the sake of comparison, the
stimulus was then delivered to skin-surface electrodes over the median nerve;
the EMG response was found to be identical.

On 12 February 1985, the Sheffield group attempted for the first time to
stimulate the human brain with a more powerful and efficient magnetic stimulator in the laboratory of P. A. Merton at the National Hospital in London.

Merton and Morton (1980) had demonstrated the feasibility of depolarizing neurons in the human motor cortex transcranially by applying direct current to the scalp. However, the technique was painful, and the possibility of achieving similar transcranial depolarization of human cortical neurons by magnetic stimulation promised the advantage of a practically painless methodology. The investigators placed an excitation coil on subjects' scalp over the motor cortex and recorded twitch muscle-action potentials from the contralateral abductor digitii minimi muscle using skin-surface electrodes. The experiment was immediately successful, with clear muscle contractions being observed in both hands without discomfort to the subjects; the first report describing stimulation of the brain was published soon thereafter in May 1985 (Barker et al., 1985).

The initial demonstration of magnetic stimulation in the motor cortex caused a groundswell of clinical and experimental interest. The first published clinical investigations using magnetic stimulation described results obtained from patients with multiple sclerosis (MS) and motor neuron disease and clearly demonstrated prolonged latencies between the motor cortex and target muscles in the MS patients (Barker et al., 1986). As the interest in TMS has grown, so has its availability. The Sheffield group introduced manufacturers to the technique in 1985, and since then stimulators have become commercially available through a number of companies. The Institute of Electrical Engineers awarded the 1987 Prize for Innovation to the Sheffield group for the development of the technique of magnetic brain stimulation. Interest in TMS has grown exponentially in the years since its creation, and clinicians and researchers worldwide are currently using magnetic brain stimulation in a wide range of applications. Indeed, the clinical neurophysiology community was quick to pick up on the importance of this discovery, and Barker's TMS soon was used widely to measure nerve conduction velocities in clinical and surgical settings (Murray, 1992; Rothwell, 1993). However, it is not in the clinical domain that TMS provides the most excitement, nor is that use the focus of our book. TMS is a tool with which to discover new facts about brain function, and it is the interface of brain activity and behavior that we seek to address. First, we need to take a look at some of the details and capabilities of a modern TMS machine.

The Nuts and Bolts of TMS

The Current Era Begins

Barker and colleagues' achievement in 1985 was to apply a magnetic pulse over the vertex of the human scalp and successfully elicit clear hand movements and accompanying EMG activity recorded from intrinsic hand muscles (Barker et al., 1985): cortical input had produced a measurable motor output. The basic, generic circuitry of magnetic stimulators is shown in figure 3.1. A capacitor charged to a high voltage is discharged into the stimulating coil via an electronic switch called a thyristor. This circuitry can be modified to produce rapid, repetitive pulses that are used in rTMS. Figure 3.2 shows the whole sequence of events in TMS from the pulse generation to cortical stimulation. The important points here are that a large current (8 kA in the example shown) is required to generate a magnetic field of sufficient intensity to stimulate the cortex and that the electric field induced in the cortex is dependent on the rate of change as well as on the intensity of the magnetic field. To achieve these requirements, the current is delivered to the coil with a very short rise time (approximately 100–200 μs) and the pulse has an overall duration of less than 1 msec. These demands also require large energy-storage capacitors and efficient energy transfer from capacitors to coil, typically in the range of 2,000 joules of stored energy

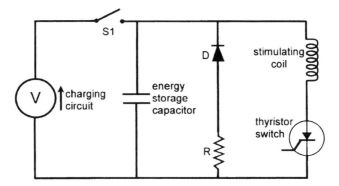

Figure 3.1   Schematic diagram of a standard (single-pulse) magnetic nerve stimulator. (From Barker, 1999, with permission.)

and 500 joules transferred to the coil in less than 100 μs. The induced field has two sources (Roth et al., 1991). One is the induction effect from the current in the coil (which is what is usually meant when discussing TMS); the other is a negligible accumulation of charge on the scalp or between the scalp and the skull. Figures 3.3 and 3.4 show the difference between two types of pulse, monophasic and biphasic, that can be produced by magnetic stimulators. The biphasic waveform employed in rTMS machines differs from the monophasic in two ways. First, in the biphasic mode up to 60% of the original energy in the pulse is returned to the capacitor, rendering rTMS more energy efficient and thus enabling the capacitors to recharge more quickly (Jalinous, 1991; Barker, 1999). More important for the end user, the biphasic waveform seems to require lower field intensities to induce a current in neural tissue (McRobbie and Foster, 1984). The reasons for the higher sensitivity of neurons to biphasic stimulation have been examined with respect to the properties of the nerve membrane (Reilly, 1992; Wada et al., 1996). The rise time of the magnetic field is important because neurons are not perfect capacitors; they are leaky, and the quicker the rise to peak intensity of the magnetic field, the less time is available for the tissue to lose charge. A fast rise time has the advantage of decreasing both the energy requirements of the stimulator and the heating of the coil (Barker, 1999).

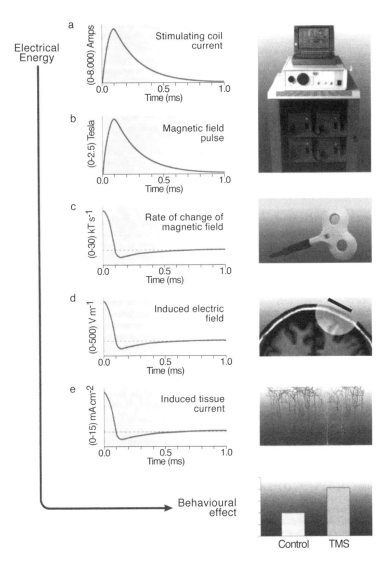

Figure 3.2   The sequence of events in TMS. An electrical current of up to 8 kA is generated by a capacitor and discharged into a circular or figure-of-eight–shaped coil, which in turn produces a magnetic pulse of up to 2 tesla. The pulse has a rise time of approximately $200~\mu$s and a duration of 1 msec and changes at a rapid rate due to its intensity and brevity. The changing magnetic field generates an electric field, resulting in neural activity or changes in resting potentials. The net change in charge density in the cortex is zero. The pulse shown here is a monophasic pulse, but in studies that require rTMS the waveform will be a train of sinewave pulses that allow repeated stimulation. (From Walsh and Cowey, 2000, with permission.)

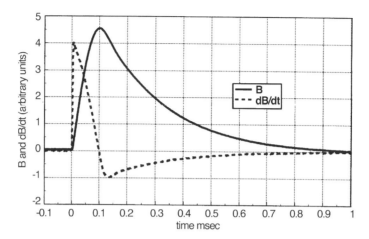

Figure 3.3   The time course of the magnetic field (B) produced by a single-pulse stimulator at the center of a stimulating coil and the resulting electrical field (dB/dt) waveform (MagStim 200 stimulator). (From Barker, 1999, with permission.)

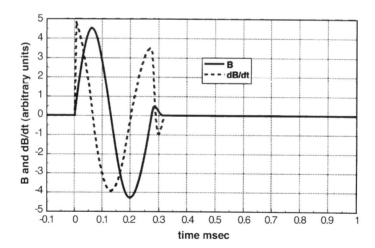

Figure 3.4   The time course of the magnetic field (B) produced by a repetitive-pulse stimulator at the center of a stimulating coil and the resulting electrical field (dB/dt) waveform (MagStim Rapid stimulator). (From Barker, 1999, with permission.)

The sequence of events shown in figure 3.2 does not answer the questions most often asked by neuropsychologists interested in using TMS to explore psychological processes: How are neurons activated? How precise is the localization? How deep can you stimulate? How long do the effects last?

HOW NEURONS ARE STIMULATED: BARKER'S ACTIVATING FUNCTIONS

In magnetic stimulation, an electric field is induced both inside and outside the axon (Nagarajan, Durand, and Warman, 1993). To produce neural activity, the induced field must differ across the cell membrane. As figure 3.5 shows, if the field is uniform with respect to the cell membrane, no current will be induced; either the axon must be bent across the electric field or the field must traverse an unbent axon. Another way of stating what is visualized in figure 3.5 is that the probability of an induced field activating a neuron is a function of the spatial derivative of the field along the nerve membrane—in Barker's words "the

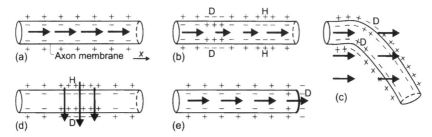

Figure 3.5   How current flow may activate neurons: schematic illustrations of activation mechanisms. In (*a*), the current flow in a uniform electric field runs parallel to a neuron and thus causes no change in transmembrane current. In (*b*), there is a gradient activation due to a nonuniform field along the axon, which causes change in transmembrane potentials, resulting in action potentials. In (*c*), the same relationship and end result is seen as in (*b*), but here the change in transmembrane current is due to spatial variation (bending) of the nerve fiber rather than inhomogeneities in the electric field. In (*d*), the depolarization is caused by transverse activation of the neuron by the induced electric field, and (*e*) represents changes in activation at the axon terminal. Regional depolarization and hyperpolarization are indicated by D and H respectively. (From Ruohonen and Ilmoniemi, 1999, with permission.)

activating function is proportional to the rate of change of the electric field" (1999; see also Reilly, 1992; Maccabee et al., 1993; Abdeen and Stuchley, 1994; Garnham, Barker, and Freeston, 1995).

The principle of the activating function can be used as a guide in thinking about the site of stimulation. Amassian et al. (1992) have modeled the stimulation of bent neurons and calculated that the excitation of straight nerves occurs near the peak electric field, whereas the activation of bent nerves occurs at the positive peak of the spatial derivative. Where the field and neuron lie in almost the same plane, presumably the spatial derivative is equivalent to the peak field. The different orientations of neurons in the cortex precludes a simple one-to-one mapping from electrical fields in homogenous conductors to the volume of neural tissue affected. Amassian gives a practical example of how knowledge of the anatomy of the cortical area being stimulated underlies accurate interpretation of the effects of TMS (figure 3.6).

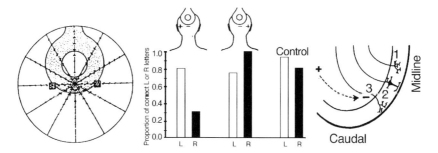

Figure 3.6   The electric field induced by TMS delivered by a round coil is modeled (*left*) in a spherical saline volume conductor. The effect on visual detection of reversing the polarity of the induced electric field is shown (*middle*), and a schematic of the possible sites of stimulation is shown (*right*). The clockwise current in the coil (*left*) induces an anticlockwise electric field, and the field intensity diminishes with distance from the peak of stimulation (center of spherical saline bath). The results from one subject show that reversing the direction of the induced field differentially suppresses visual performance in the left or right visual hemifield (Amassian et al., 1994). The most likely point of stimulation (*right*) is the bend in the axon (3). Excitation of the axonal arborizations (1) is less likely due to relative high resitance; excitation of the dendritic arbors (2) is less likely due to relative reduced electrical excitability (Reilly, 1989). (From Amassian et al., 1998, with permission.)

EXCITATION, INHIBITION—IT'S ALL "NOISE"

A frequently asked question is whether TMS has excitatory or inhibitory effects in the cortex. The question arises because TMS can induce movements or phosphenes, but it also can have disruptive, "inhibitory" effects on perceptual or motor performance. If one considers the mechanisms of TMS induction (described earlier), it becomes readily apparent that TMS cannot be expected to distinguish between excitatory and inhibitory neurons within a region of stimulation, nor can it be expected to distinguish between orthodromic and antidromic direction of stimulation. Delivery of a TMS pulse will randomly excite neurons that lie within the effective induced electrical field. For these reasons, it is best to consider TMS as operating in two ways. In its disruptive mode, the mode of most interest to psychologists and the one on which this book concentrates, TMS applied while a subject is trying to perform a task induces neural noise into the signal-processing system. Just as the stimulation is likely to be random with respect to inhibition, excitation and direction of current along any given membrane, so, too, can it be presumed to be random with respect to the organization of the neural assemblies involved in any particular task. There are other situations in which TMS might be considered to operate in a productive mode and to add signal rather than noise—for example, in the functional enhancements produced by TMS (Walsh et al., 1998b) or in the production of phosphenes (Kammer, 1999; Kammer and Nusseck, 1998). However, the enhancements reported by Walsh et al. were caused by a disruption in one area resulting in disinhibition in a competing region of cortex, and as Kammer has argued cogently, the physiological effects that produce phosphenes are identical with those that produce visual deficits. We show later that these outcomes also might be the product of neural noise (see chapter 4).

COILS AND NEURONS

The two types of coil in most common use are circular and figure-of-eight in shape, and the regions of effective stimulation produced by these two configurations depend on the geometry of the coil and of the neurons underlying the coil and on local conduction variability. Figure 3.7 (plate 1) shows the distribution of an induced electric field under a round coil (*top*), and figure 3.8 (plate 2) (*top*) shows the distribution of the spatial derivative of the field with respect to a straight axon that will be hyperpolarized at B and polarized at A ("virtual anode" and "virtual cathode," respectively, in Barker's terminology). Nerves lying tangential to any other part of the coil will be similarly stimulated. This does not mean that the effects of TMS are restricted to the cortical area located precisely under the windings of the coil. The neurons receiving stimulation will activate their neighbors and also affect the organization of other interacting pairs of neurons. With this round coil, specificity of the area stimulated can be increased by making contact between only one arc of the coil and the scalp.

The side of the coil with which stimulation is applied also will affect the outcome. With a monophasic pulse, the current travels clockwise with respect to one face of the coil and counterclockwise with respect to the other. This disposition can be used to bias stimulation in one or other direction and has been used to stimulate selectively one or other hemisphere while apparently stimulating in the midline (Amassian et al., 1994; Meyer et al., 1991) and to enhance the efficacy of motor cortex stimulation by applying the current direction optimal for stimulation of that region (Brasil-Neto et al., 1992a,c).

Stimulation with a figure-of-eight coil increases the focality of stimulation (Ueno, Tashiro, and Harada, 1988). This configuration is of two circular coils that carry current in opposite directions, and, where the coils meet, there is a summation of the electric field. Figures 3.7 (bottom) and 3.8 (bottom) show the induced electric field and the rate of change of the field with respect to a straight neuronal axon. In addition to the new "summated" anode and cathode produced by the figure-of-eight coil, the two separate windings maintain their ability to induce a field under the outer parts of the windings. However, in experiments where the center of the figure eight is placed over the region of interest, the outer parts of the coil are usually several centimeters away from the scalp and thus unlikely to induce effective fields, therefore increasing the probability that stimulation will be relatively focal: But how focal (figure 3.9)?

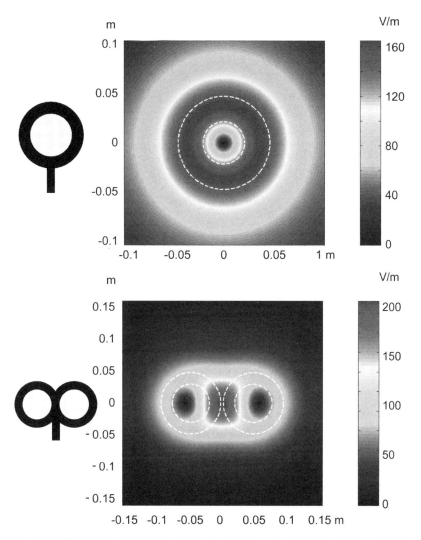

Figure 3.7   Distribution of the induced electric fields by a circular (*top*) and figure-of-eight (*bottom*) stimulating coil. The circular coil has 41.5 mm inside-turn diameter, 91.5 mm outside turn diameter (mean 66.5 mm), and fifteen turns of copper wire. The figure-of-eight coil has 56 mm inside-turn diameter, 90 mm outside-turn diameter (mean 73 mm), and nine turns of copper wire on each wing. The outline of each coil is depicted with dashed white lines on the representation of the induced fields. The electric field amplitude is calculated in a plane 20 mm below a realistic model of the coil ($dI/dt = 10^8$ A s^{-1}). (Figure created by Anthony Barker, used with permission.) See plate 1 for color version.

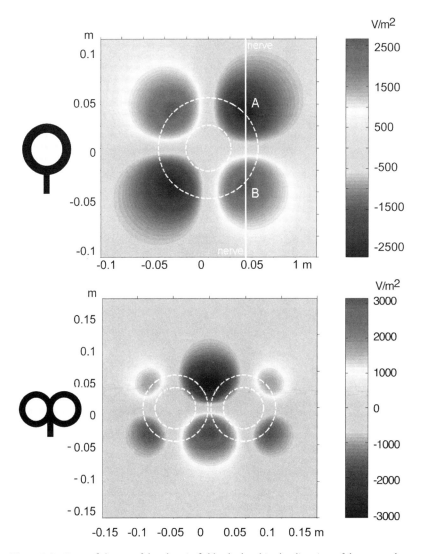

Figure 3.8   Rate of change of the electric field calculated in the direction of the nerve along the axis AB, measured in the same plane as coils shown in figure 3.7. (Figure created by Anthony Barker, used with permission.) See plate 2 for color version.

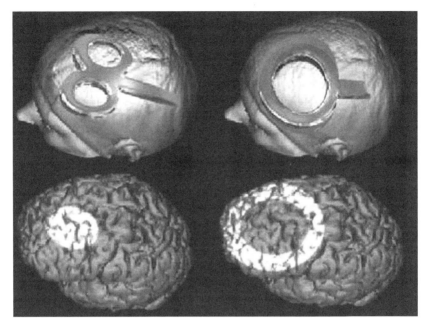

Figure 3.9   Cartoon-like representation of the markedly different brain regions targeted by TMS using a circular or figure-of-eight–shaped coil centered over the same scalp position. Given the differences in induced fields, the results of an experiment done with the figure-of-eight–shaped coil may not be reproducible with a circular coil centered over the same brain region because different brain areas would be affected.

HOW FOCAL IS TMS?

From the foregoing discussion, one might be forgiven for thinking it impossible to target specific cortical areas with TMS. Several converging lines of evidence now show that there is good reason for confidence in the anatomical focality and, more important, in the functional focality of TMS. One could simply appeal to the surface validity of TMS—Barker's first demonstration of motor cortex stimulation, for example, was strongly suggestive of relatively selective, suprathreshold stimulation of the hand area of the cortex. Perhaps there was some spread of current to arm, shoulder, and face regions of the motor cortex, but in the absence of movements from these parts of the body one must infer that the stimulation was *effectively* precise—that is, stimulation of the other areas was subthreshold for producing a behavioral effect. There are many other examples of surface validity: Phosphenes are more likely if the coil is placed over the visual cortex (Marg, 1991; Meyer et al., 1991; Kastner, Demmer, and Ziemann, 1998; Kammer, 1999); speech arrest more likely if stimulation is applied over facial motor or frontal cortex (Pascual-Leone et al., 1991b,c; Epstein et al., 1996; Stewart et al., 2001a); and neglect and extinction-like deficits more likely if the coil targets the parietal lobe (Pascual-Leone et al., 1994; Ashbridge, Walsh, and Cowey, 1997; Fierro et al., 2000). Mapping of the motor cortex with EMG-recorded responses also shows discrete representations of the fingers, hand, arm, face, trunk, and legs in a pattern that matches the gross organization of the motor homunculus (Wasserman et al., 1992; Singh et al., 1997), sensitive both to coil location and intensity (Brasil-Neto et al., 1992a,c).

There are more direct measures of the specificity of TMS. Wassermann et al. (1996) mapped the cortical representation of a hand muscle with TMS and coregistered the inferred volumetric fields with anatomical MRIs from each subject and with PET images obtained while subjects moved the finger that had been mapped with TMS. In all subjects, the estimated fields induced by TMS met the surface of the brain at the anterior lip of the central sulcus and extended along the precentral gyrus for a few millimeters anterior to the central sulcus. When compared with the PET activations, the MRI locations were all within 5 to 22 mm—an impressive correspondence across three techniques. A similarly impressive level of correspondence has been seen in other studies that have correlated TMS with fMRI (Terao et al., 1998b) and with MEG (Morioka et al., 1995b; Ruohonen et al., 1996). There are reasons for caution in interpreting these data (see Wasserman et al., 1996); for example, the hand area activated lies deep in the central sulcus, possibly too deep to be activated directly by TMS and therefore presumably is activated trans-synaptically. The evidence for trans-synaptic actvation comes from a comparison of the EMG latencies elicited by electrical or magnetic stimulation (Day et al., 1987, 1989a,b; Amassian et al.,

1990). Magnetically evoked latencies are approximately 1–2 msec longer than electrically evoked ones, which can be explained on the basis of which neurons are most likely to be stimulated by each technique (Rothwell, 1994). TMS is more likely to stimulate neurons that run parallel to the cortical surface, whereas electrical stimulation can directly stimulate pyramidal output neurons that run orthogonal to the cortical surface. Thus, the 1–2 msec delay between electrical and magnetic cortical stimulation may be accounted for by the time taken for the stimulation to be transmitted from the interneurons to the pyramidal cells.

Knowledge of which kinds of cells are stimulated based on temporal information can inform the interpretation of functional specificity. A clear example comes from the work of Heinen and colleagues (1998), who measured central motor-conduction time (CCT) by recording TMS-evoked EMG responses from the first dorsal interosseous muscle of children (mean age seven years) and adults (mean age twenty-nine years) in relaxed and facilitated (i.e., hand tensed) conditions. The adults' relaxed latencies were significantly shorter (by approximately 2 msec) than the children's, but there was no difference between the two groups in the facilitated condition. This relative difference between relaxed and facilitated CCT is attributed to the temporal summation of descending corticospinal volleys at the alpha motoneuron (Hess, Mills, and Murray, 1986; Chiappa et al., 1991). Heinen et al. hypothesized, therefore, that the difference between the adults and children was "due to an immature synaptic organization at either the first or the second neuron of the pyramidal tract" (1998)—a level of resolution that warns against confusing the apparent physical resolution of a technique with the intellectual resolution possible when using it.

Other evidence strengthens the correlation between targeted and activated cortical regions. Paus and colleagues (1997, 1998, 1999) have carried out a number of studies in which TMS has been combined with analysis of PET activations using a method of frameless stereotaxy that aligns MRI landmarks and the center of the stimulating coil with an accuracy within 0.4 to 0.8 cm. The first critical finding of these experiments is that TMS has a major effect approximately under the center of a figure-of-eight coil and secondary effects at sites that are known to be anatomically connected (figure 3.10). The second finding

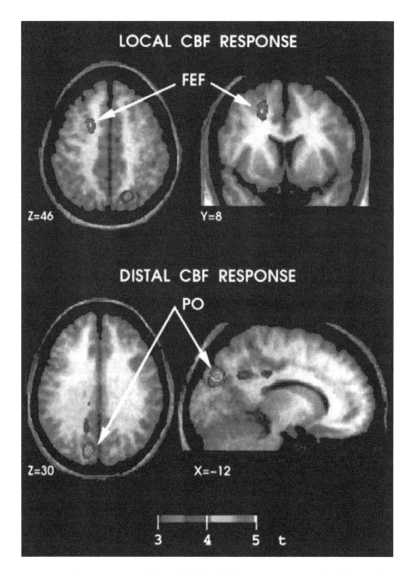

Figure 3.10   Changes in regional cerebral blood flow (rCBF) as a result of TMS. The top figure shows a significant correlation between TMS and rCBF in the vicinity of the frontal eye fields (FEFs), the regions targeted by the TMS pulses. The bottom figure shows one of the cortical regions that most likely was activated through spread of stimulation effects, namely the parieto-occipital (PO) cortex of the ipsilateral hemisphere—a region similar to that known to be connected with the FEF in monkeys. (From Paus et al., 1997, with permission.)

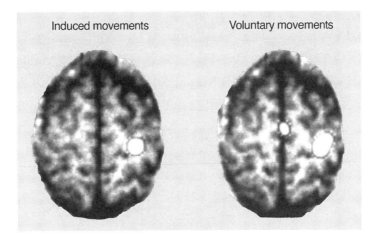

Figure 3.11   The spatial and functional specificity of TMS is evident in the correspondence between changes in blood flow induced by TMS over the motor cortex to produce a finger movement and the activity produced by intentional or voluntary movement, which also produces SMA activity. (From Siebner et al., 1998, with permission.)

is that optimal stimulation depends critically on the precise orientation of the coil (see also Hill, Davey, and Kennard, 2000; Kammer et al., 2001).

Further evidence of the accuracy of TMS is seen in figure 3.11. Siebner and colleagues (1998) compared the changes in regional cerebral blood flow caused by 2 Hz rTMS over the motor cortex, at an intensity sufficient to elicit an arm movement, with blood flow changes caused by the actual movement of the arm. The correspondence was striking. TMS-induced movements and voluntary movements both activated primary sensorimotor cortex (SM1; area 4) ipsilateral to the site of stimulation. Voluntary movement also activated the ipsilateral supplementary motor area (SMA) (area 6), and the motor activity associated with the voluntary movement was more extensive than that elicited by rTMS. This difference could be because the voluntary arm movement was slightly greater than the TMS movement or because voluntary activity involves more muscles than TMS activity. Whatever the difference, it is a clear example of the specificity of TMS and of the physiological validity of TMS effects.

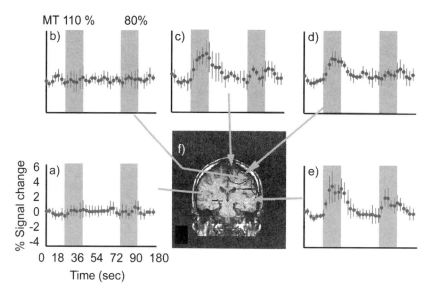

Figure 3.12   Time activity curves of a subject's brain during rest and with TMS over the thumb representation of the motor cortex. These data were obtained by interleaving BOLD fMRI and TMS. The TMS was given at 1 Hz for 8 sec. The spatial and temporal resolution of the measurements are approximately 2 mm and 3 sec. (From Bohning et al., 1999, with permission.)

Further evidence comes from studies of TMS effects measured by fMRI by George, Bohning, and their colleagues. The importance of the technical achievement of combining TMS and fMRI is discussed in chapter 9, but here the important point is, as in Siebner and colleagues' study, the remarkable correspondence between the motor cortex activation produced by real and TMS-induced movements (figure 3.12). These studies are important examples of the spatial specificity of TMS. They do not mean that the induced electric field is limited to the functional units stimulated, nor do they suggest that activation of neurons is limited to the areas seen in PET and fMRI, but they show unequivocally that the theoretical spread of the induced field is not the determinant of the area of effective stimulation and that the functional localization of TMS is to a significant degree under experimenter control.

Some of the confusion over the functional specificity of TMS is matched by the apparent specificity of other techniques with which TMS is sometimes compared. Given a coil placed on the scalp with the intention of stimulating the motor cortex, we can say with complete confidence that we will be able to stimulate an unknown number of different kinds of neurons in the vicinity of the motor cortex. With an electrode placed stereotactically in the brain of a rat, we can do much better, but there are still severe constraints. Ranck makes the point with precision: "The phrase 'electrical stimulation of the lateral hypothalamus' is a shortened version of the statement that 'there was a stimulating electrode in the lateral hypothalamus which affected an unknown number and unknown kinds of cells at unknown locations in the vicinity of the electrode" (1975). Ranck's general point applies to all techniques that either record from or stimulate neural assemblies. The question is how to interpret the meaning of the stimulation results. Ranck advised that the best way was to understand the activity of single cells and exhorted his colleagues to "think cellular." In magnetic stimulation experiments, the appropriate level of analysis is not prescribed so readily. If the hypothesis and the knowledge of the system under investigation are sufficient, one can think cellular (cf. Heinen et al., 1998). In most neurocognitive experiments and in the experiments discussed throughout this book, thinking cellular is not an option other than to compare effects with the known properties of neurons from intra- and extracellular recording studies or to combine TMS with pharmacological manipulations.

Studies of EEG responses by Ilmoniemi and colleagues (1997) provide another demonstration of the relative primary and secondary specificity of TMS. As figure 3.13 shows, stimulation over the visual or motor cortex elicits EEG responses around the site of stimulation in the first few milliseconds after TMS. Within 20–30 msec, this activity is mirrored by a secondary area of activity in the homotopic regions of the contralateral hemisphere. These delays in homotopic areas are a rich source of hypotheses regarding the timing of effects in interhemispheric interactions (see chapter 5). The utility and specificity of this combination of techniques was demonstrated further by applying TMS to the motor cortex of a patient who had suffered a lesion to the right basal ganglia

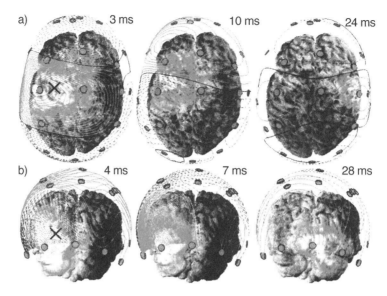

Figure 3.13   Dynamics of changes in neural activity induced by TMS. Four milliseconds after TMS over the occipital lobe, most of the electrical activity recorded with high-resolution EEG is around the area directly under the TMS stimulation site (marked by the X). By 7 msec, this activity has spread to the midline, and by 28 msec there is clearly contralateral activation. (From Ilmoniemi et al., 1997, with permission.)

and had lost fine finger control in his left hand and some control of his left arm. When the intact hemisphere was stimulated, EEG responses were seen in the motor cortex of both hemispheres. When the motor cortex ipsilateral to the affected basal ganglia was stimulated, some EEG response was seen ipsilaterally, but none was transmitted interhemispherically to the intact hemisphere.

DEPTH OF STIMULATION

The depth of penetration of TMS is another important question, and, as with the question of lateral specificity, there is no easy answer, but again there are good reasons to think that the approximations available are meaningful and can

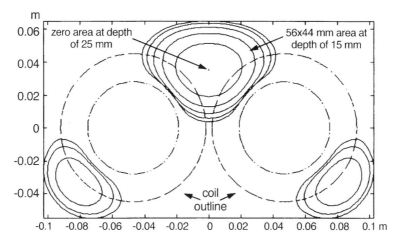

Figure 3.14   Estimated stimulation areas at depth intervals of 5 mm beginning at the cortical surface. (From Barker, 1999, with permission.)

be used to guide interpretation of results. Models of the electric field at different depths from the coil suggest that relatively wide areas are stimulated close to the coil, decreasing in surface area as the field is measured at distances farther from the coil. The image offered by these models is of an egg-shaped cone, with the apex, which marks the point of the smallest area of stimulation, farthest from the coil. This is a result of an interaction between the decrease in magnetic field strength and a progressive loss of focality. For a standard figure–eight coil, one estimate is that stimulation 5 mm below the coil will cover an area of approximately 7 by 6 cm. This area decreases to 4 by 3 cm at 20 mm below the coil—that is, in the region of the cortical surface (figure 3.14). Calculations of induced electric fields as a function of depth also can be used as a guide to specificity because stimulation at points where the fields overlap allows subtraction of the effects. If the coil positioned at the central site in figure 3.15 disrupts performance on a behavioral task, the effective site of stimulation can be said to be anywhere within, around, or connected to the neurons crossed by the field. If stimulation at the sites on either side fails to disrupt the task, then the overlap in

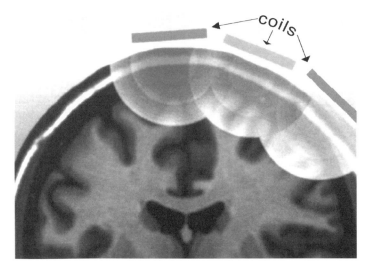

Figure 3.15 The subtraction of spatial effects in TMS. From models of TMS-induced electrical fields, one can infer the region of stimulation. By stimulating at neighboring regions on the scalp, one can refine the these inferences and, notwithstanding the uncertainty of any one field, can make reasonable functional anatomical attributions. The "coils" and induced fields in this figure are illustrative of the methodolgical rationale and do not represent real configurations and effects. (From Walsh and Cowey, 2000, with permission.)

fields between the central and either of the two lateral sites can be said to be in-effective regions of the field, and the most effective field is the central subregion. So our notion of the effective resolution of TMS can be refined: whereas a sin-gle pulse of TMS cannot be said to have a small, volumetric resolution in the cortex, from a functional point of view it can be shown to have a small scalp res-olution and an inferred or subtracted volumetric resolution when multiple sites are compared. A comparison might be made here with fMRI and, say, a cortical area such as visual area V5 (Watson et al., 1993); it is clearly not the case that moving visual stimuli activate V5 alone. Rather, the specificity of this area is in-ferred, quite properly, by subtracting the activations caused by stationary or col-ored stimuli or different kinds of visual motion.

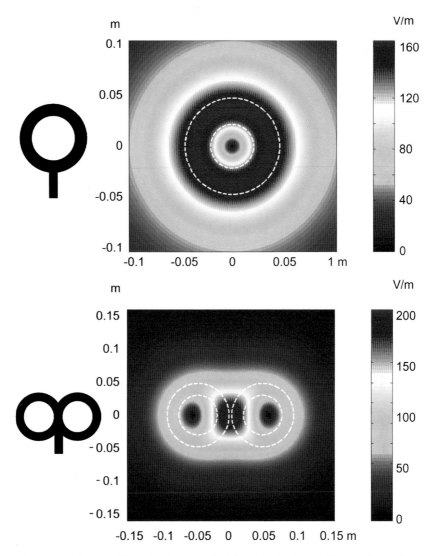

Plate 1 Distribution of the induced electric fields by a circular (*top*) and figure–of–eight (*bottom*) stimulating coil. The circular coil has 41.5 mm inside–turn diameter, 91.5 mm outside–turn diameter (mean 66.5 mm) and fifteen turns of copper wire. The figure–of–eight coil has five 6 mm inside–turn diameter, 90 mm outside–turn diameter (mean 73 mm), and nine turns of copper wire on each wing. The outline of each coil is depicted with dashed white lines on the representation of the induced fields. The electric field amplitude is calculated in a plane 20 mm below a realistic model of the coil ($dI/dt = 10^8$ A s^{-1}). (Figure created by Anthony Barker; used with permission.) See chapter 3.

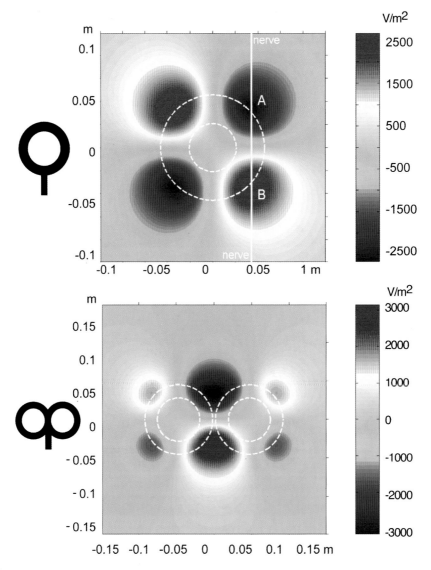

Plate 2 Rate of change of the electric field calculated in the direction of the nerve along the axis AB, measured in the same plane as coils shown in plate 1. (Figure created by Anthony Barker, used with permission.) See chapter 3.

THE TEMPORAL WINDOW OF TMS

The cycle of a single pulse of TMS is approximately 1 msec (figure 3.2), which determines the temporal resolution of the application of TMS. The duration of the effect in the cortex is difficult to determine because the neurons stimulated by the field may take time to recover their normal functional state and normal interactions with other cells. Several TMS studies have applied single-pulse TMS at intervals of 10 msec and obtained effects that suggest that TMS can distinguish processes within such a small time window, but the time window is probabilistic rather than fixed. Figure 3.16 illustrates how the time window is constructed. First, the effect of TMS is likely to be an ON step function or at least a steep ramp function because many fibers will be stimulated simultaneously. However, the offset of the effects are likely to be a shallow ramp function because fibers of different sizes and at different orientations will be affected to different degrees and will recover at different rates. As the population of neurons recovers, the neural noise added to the system diminishes. If one also assumes a finite period during which the area stimulated is critical to the task and that this criticality is also probabilistic, then the degree to which TMS will interfere with processing is a function of the noise induced at any time T and the probability that the neurons in that area are involved in the task.

SAFETY

Beware of an optimist wielding a stimulating coil.

—*R. Jalinous, Guide to Magnetic Stimulation*

The use of TMS is rightly subject to approval by local ethical committees, and some precautions must be taken in all studies using the technique. The safety of single-pulse TMS is well established, but further precautions should be taken when using rTMS. The magnetic field produced by stimulating coils can cause a loud noise, and temporary elevations in auditory thresholds have been

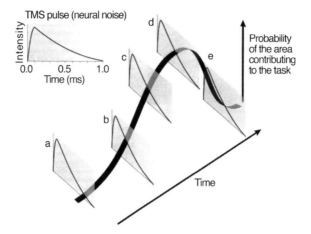

Figure 3.16 A probabilistic picture of the relationship between pulse strength and behavioral effects. The upper portion of the figure shows that the intensity of the TMS pulse is greatest close to the time of onset and then declines within 1 msec. The effect this pattern has on behavior is a function of the intensity of the physiological effects of TMS and the probability that the neurons stimulated are critical to the task. The pulse at (*a*) would not have a behavioral effect because it is applied too early. The pulse at (*b*) would interfere with behavior because an early (i.e., high) phase of the TMS noise is applied even though the probability (P) of the area's involvement is low. Similarly, (*c*) and (*d*) would have a behavioral effect because of the high P of the area's involvement when the pulse is delivered. The pulses applied at (*c*) and (*e*) arrive at similar P values in the area's function, but the neural noise induced is higher at (*e*) because there is no recovery time. Thus, the product of neural noise times neural necessity would be higher at (*e*) than at (*c*). This way of thinking about the time course of TMS effects shows that the temporal resolution of TMS is limited by two factors (duration of TMS pulse effects and duration of an area's involvement in the task). The figure, viewed in a conceptually different manner, also provides a clear illustration of why TMS effects should not correspond to the peaks of ERP or MEG times. The appropriate application of TMS may well be able to have effects at times well before (*b*) and (*c*) or well after (*e*), the reported peak. (From Walsh and Cowey, 2000, with permission.)

reported (Pascual-Leone et al., 1993c). The use of ear plugs is recommended in all experiments. Some subjects may experience headaches or nausea or may simply find the face twitches and other peripheral effects of TMS too uncomfortable. Such subjects obviously should be released from any obligation to continue the experiments. More serious are the concerns that TMS may induce an epileptic seizure. In a number of cases, rTMS did induce epileptic fits, and caution is necessary. As a guide in experimentation, any subject with any personal or family history of epilepsy or other neurological condition should be precluded from taking part in an experiment that does not involve investigation of that condition. Pascual-Leone et al. (1993c) assessed the safety of rTMS and noted that seizures could be induced in subjects who had no identifiable, preexisting risk factors. The paper presents some guidelines for the use of rTMS, so familiarity with this paper should be a prerequisite of using rTMS. However, the paper is not exhaustive; it is based on only three sites of stimulation and expresses pulse intensity as a percentage of *motor* threshold. It recently has been argued that studies that apply rTMS to areas other than the motor cortex cannot simply lift stimulation parameters and criteria based on motor cortex excitability and assume they transfer to other conditions. There is no necessary relationship between motor cortex excitability and that of other cortical regions (Stewart, Walsh, and Rothwell, 2001). It is also recommended that anyone wishing to use rTMS visit the TMS Web site (http://pni.unibe.ch/maillist.htm). The TMS community is constantly reviewing safety procedures, and this Web site is a starting point for access to sound information (although much of it is directed to a clinical psychiatry audience). A more recent paper (Wassermann, 1998) summarizes the prevailing views that exist within the TMS community, as expressed at a meeting in 1996. The adverse effects recorded include seizures, though they are rare; some enhancement effects on motor reaction time and verbal recall; and effects on affect (some subjects have been reported to cry and others to laugh following application of rTMS to the left prefrontal cortex). There is little information about potential longer-term problems with rTMS, but the issue cannot be ducked. If, on the one hand, rTMS is potentially useful in the alleviation of depression (Pascual-Leone et al., 1996; George et al., 1995, 1996), it must be conceded that it can have longer-term effects. It would be disingenuous to suggest that all long-term effects are likely to be beneficial rather than deleterious. It should be noted, however, that improvements in mood do follow several sessions of magnetic stimulation, and the effects appear to be cumulative. A simple precaution that may be taken is to prevent individual subjects from taking part in repeated experiments over a short period of time. The use of rTMS should follow a close reading of Pascual-Leone et al.'s (1993c) and Wassermann's (1998) reports. Studies of neuropsychological functions, such as those discussed throughout this book, seldom even approach the safety limits, and if one follows the guide given in chapter 4, it will be a simple matter to design experiments that use minimal intensities and durations of TMS.

A concern sometimes raised about TMS is that it is in some sense "unnatural" to apply magnetic pulses to people's scalps because the resulting neural activity is "abnormal" and may have long-term consequences. If ecological accuracy were a requirement of psychological experiments, one wonders how spatial frequency gratings, stroop stimuli, adaptation experiments (the McCullough effect, for example, can last for months), and many other manipulations can be justified. But the question is still important: If we are to understand the mechanisms of TMS, we need to know how the neural noise induced can be compared with real neural activity and with the functional noise introduced in dual-task experiments and in other psychological interference techniques. An understanding of how the cortex responds to TMS is also critical to the interpretation of longer-term effects of TMS and to accurate analysis of experiments in which TMS is combined with fMRI.

Niehaus et al. (1999) have approached this question using transcranial doppler sonography (TCD, a noninvasive technique that allows blood flow, as velocities, to be recorded from intracranial arteries [see Bogdahn, 1998]) to observe rapid changes in the hemodynamic response to TMS and to compare this response with "real" sensory (in this case, visual) stimulation. As figure 3.17 shows, TMS produced changes in blood flow that occurred earlier and were larger in the hemisphere ipsilateral to stimulation over the occipital lobe (cf. the results of Ilmoniemi et al., 1997). There was also a close correspondence between blood flow associated with trains of 5 Hz TMS and 5 Hz light flicker (figure 3.18), thus supporting the assumption that blood-flow changes evoked by TMS are a reflection of neural activity rather than nonspecific effects on the vascular system. It is important to note that there were no long-term changes associated with the use of rTMS.

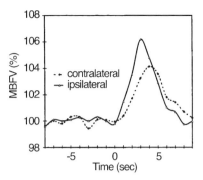

Figure 3.17   The cerebral haemodynamic response to TMS over the motor cortex in ten subjects. Five trains of 10 Hz were given to each subject. Time-locked average mean blood flow volume (MBFV) changes in the middle cerebral artery ipsilateral and contralateral to the stimulation site is shown. (From Niehuas et al., 1999, with permission.)

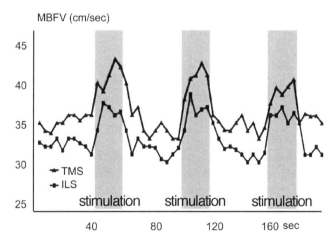

Figure 3.18   Changes in MBFV in the left posterior cerebral artery during rTMS over the left occipital cortex or during visual stimulation with light flicker. Stimulation was performed with rTMS trains of 5 Hz and 20 sec duration and intermittent light stimulation (ILS) with the same frequency and stimulation duration.

Creating Virtual Patients: A Guide to Mechanism and Methodology

What Is a Virtual Lesion?

The first use of the virtual-lesion methodology in the motor system was by Day et al. (1989a,b), who applied single-pulse TMS to the motor cortex while subjects carried out a simple instruction to flex or extend their wrist. The subjects were given an auditory "go" signal, followed 100 msec later by the TMS pulse and therefore before the predicted onset of voluntary EMG activity, which occurred 30–40 msec later. The effect of the TMS was to markedly increase reaction time (RT) to flex or extend the wrist. This apparently simple experiment contains the seeds of some of the most important principles in understanding the effects of TMS.

The choice of dependent variable in a TMS experiment depends on the function to be disrupted, but reaction time is proving to be a more versatile dependent measure than error rates (see later in this chapter). This may reflect the kinds of experiments being carried out in this first wave of cognitive TMS experiments, and new paradigms may be more successful with errors as the dependent measure. In most experiments to date, single-pulse TMS causes RT increases more often than errors, and the increases are frequently longer than 50 msec. It is as if the brain has been "put on hold" for tens of milliseconds. In the Day et al. experiment reaction times were elevated by up to 150 msec (mean 64 msec) in a task with a mean reaction time of only 136 msec (figure 4.1). Day et al. also varied the intensity of the stimulus and found that the EMG latency increased as a function of TMS intensity (figure 4.2). The mechanism of the delaying effect may have been caused by abolition of some part of the motor program, which had to be recalculated when the neural assembly disrupted had recovered. Day et al. argued that the most likely explanation is that the TMS inhibited "transmission of information through a central process. . . . [And] these cells would be unresponsive until they had recovered from the inhibitory process" (1989, 660–661). The fact that increasing stimulator output intensity produced longer delays suggests that TMS can disrupt a function by stimulating a subset of the neurons critical to a task and that the more of this subset is stimulated, the longer the recovery period lasts. But what happens to the information that is disrupted? It is not lost, but it seems equally unlikely that it is stored somewhere until the TMS disruption ceases.

In chapter 3, we described a probabilistic account of how TMS can induce sufficient current to delay processing in a task. This model also provides an operational explanation of how a virtual lesion acts as "neural noise" in the same way as adding visual noise to a display causes subjects to take longer to identify the stimulus. Two such examples are difficult visual search tasks, wherein every additional distractor increases reaction time, and motion coherence thresholds (or any threshold measure, in fact) wherein the time taken to make a response increases as one approaches the limits of detection or discrimination. There would be no suggestion here that transmission of information is blocked or stored pending the recovery of the visual system. Rather, the visual system is carrying out its normal function in trying to complete a signal detection analysis. Under most conditions, TMS adds only enough noise to delay the process, but if the task is difficult enough (i.e., in circumstances where internal noise is already high) and the magnetic stimulation intensity high enough, errors can occur. Psychologists understand this mechanism very well; they have been using it for decades in the form of dual tasks and masking, but the whole point of these

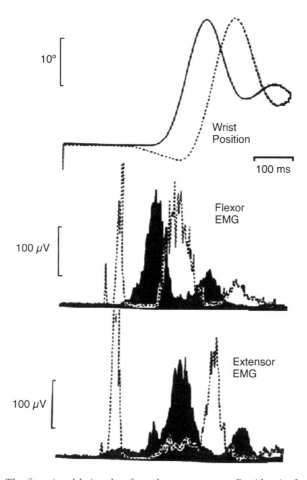

Figure 4.1 The first virtual-lesion data from the motor system. Rapid wrist-flexion movements in a single subject in response to an audio signal given at the start of the EMG sweep, with (dotted lines) and without (solid lines) TMS applied 100 msec after the start of the recording. The upper two traces show the average wrist positions, the middle traces the EMG activity recorded from the flexor muscle, and the lower trace EMG activity from the extensor. The control movement is characterized by alternating bursts of activity in flexors and extensors (compare dark regions in middle and lower traces). When TMS was applied (70% of stimulator output), the activity follows the same alternating pattern but is delayed by approximately 60 msec. The activity near the beginning of the middle and lower traces (approximately 15 msec after TMS pulse delivery) is the TMS stimulus artifact, which in this subject produced a small extension movement. (From Day et al., 1989b, with permission.)

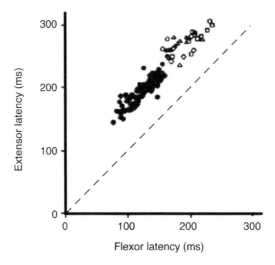

Figure 4.2   The effects of TMS intensity on reaction time. The latency (measured from the audio signal) to onset of wrist-flexor (agonist) EMG activity plotted against the onset or wrist-extensor (antagonist) EMG activity for individual trials of a series of wrist flexion movements made by one subject. Control trials are indicated by closed circles, and trials with an interposed TMS pulse given 60 msec after the tone at different intensities of stimulation are shown by open symbols (open circles denote 60%, triangles 70%, and squares 80% of stimulator output). The delay in onset of EMG activity in the forearm muscles produced by each stimulus during wrist flexion is similar for both flexor and extensor muscle groups and increases with higher intensities of stimulation. (From Day et al., 1989b, with permission.)

experiments is to add noise selectively to one processing system until performance breaks down (see Pashler, 1998).

At this stage, then, a virtual lesion can be defined as a means of adding neural noise to a task. This still raises the question of how one might resolve the temporal resolution of the virtual lesion with the temporal information from EEG or MEG studies. One of the features of single-pulse TMS studies (see chapter 5) is that the critical time of applying the pulse seems to be earlier than the time of critical differences in ERP studies and closer to the latencies observed in single-unit studies. One reason this might be the case is that TMS can have an effect at any stage in the development of an ERP waveform—at the evolution, the peak, or the tail, during any of which times critical processes may be occurring in the area stimulated. It is still not clear for how long the TMS pulse actually destabilizes neural processing, but in principle a long-lasting effect can have a small time window of efficacy coupled with a large effect on time taken to perform a task. Neither the ERP nor TMS can indicate exactly when the onset of the critical process occurs, but it is clear that the critical TMS times are closer to doing so. As we saw in chapter 3, although a TMS pulse has a definite duration, it is reasonable to assume that the size of the effect (i.e., the induced neural noise) peaks at onset of the pulse and diminishes throughout the duration of the effect. Evidence supporting this notion is that whereas TMS effects do not correlate well with ERPs, they do correspond to single-unit data (e.g., Corthout et al., 1999b; Ashbridge et al., 1997).

Some caution should be exercised regarding the correspondence between the times at which TMS has an effect and timing information from other methodologies. Some studies do show a close correspondence between ERP and TMS times (e.g., Zangaladze et al., 1999) or between MEG and TMS times (Ganis et al., 2000), but the number of studies that have compared different techniques with exactly the same stimulus and response conditions is very small, and it is too soon to say whether one should expect a constant relationship between recording techniques and TMS interference times or whether the relationship is mutable depending on how TMS causes disruption in any given task and on which neural generators are the source of the ERP or MEG information. There is no direct evidence yet, after all, that the signals disrupted by TMS are those measured by ERPs.

The definition of a virtual lesion can be refined now to a means of adding neural noise to a task at a stage of processing that may be earlier than the onset of the critical operations due to the lifespan of the neural disruption. Yet another question arises, however. If TMS acts as a virtual lesion by disrupting organized neural firing, how can TMS lead to enhancements rather than deficits on some tasks (see "Facilitations: Beware of False Profits" in this chapter)?

SOME GUIDANCE ON EXPERIMENTAL PROCEDURE

To do a TMS experiment, one needs to know where to stimulate, when to stimulate, and at what intensity, rate, and duration. The answers to these questions will differ from experiment to experiment and may change even during the experiment as unexpected effects emerge and preconceptions are confounded; single-unit physiologists and psychologists testing patients will be familiar with this feeling. To provide a framework for working through experimental considerations, we discuss here a "perfect" mosaic of experiments that together contain the kernel of all the major methodological elements it is important to discuss. The composite experiments we discuss concern mainly studies of cortical visual area V5, which shows considerable specialization for the analysis of visual motion (Watson et al., 1993). We also consider some aspects of stimulation of the motor cortex. For each part of these experiments, we discuss the reasoning behind the method of localization chosen and the stimulation parameters used. The theoretical importance of these studies is discussed in detail in the relevant chapters later in the book, but here the aim is to provide a first stop for anyone wishing to embark on a program of TMS studies; thus, the emphasis is on the methodology. All of the experiments we discuss used normal, neurologically intact adults; they do not cover every eventuality or details of stimulating children or neurological patients.

WHEN, WHERE, AND HOW LONG TO STIMULATE

To study the role of V5 in human motion perception, one needs to be able to target the correct area. The method of choice would be to carry out a motion-perception study using fMRI, to locate the scalp area overlying the area identified as V5, and to apply TMS at that point. A clear illustration of this method is shown in figure 4.3. Pascual-Leone et al. applied TMS over V5 at 120% of motor threshold at 10 Hz for up to 2 sec and reduced accuracy on a motion coherence task. As the figure-of-eight coil was moved away from this site in steps of 1 cm, the detection performance improved. The stimulation parameters were selected

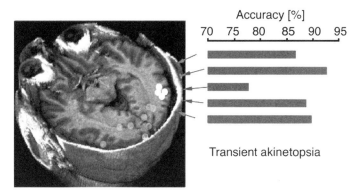

Figure 4.3   Activations from a BOLD fMRI study show the regions associated with presentation of visual motion displays. Repetitive-pulse TMS was applied with a TMS coil at 120% of motor threshold, at 10 Hz for a maximum of 2 sec at points around the areas of maximum activity in an attempt to disrupt motion perception. The bar histogram depicts the subject's mean accuracy in the detection of the direction of random motion during TMS to five scalp areas. Note the significant decline in performance limited to the scalp location of the coil overlying the motion-perception "hotspot" in the fMRI. (From Pascual-Leone, Bartres-Faz, and Keenan, 1999, with permission.)

for several reasons. The intensity of the stimulation was selected on the basis of known safety parameters (see chapter 3), and the authors opted to use 10 Hz because they were testing a functional localization hypothesis and not a timing hypothesis, which would have required single-pulse TMS. The duration of the stimulation, which began at stimulus onset, ensured that the critical period of processing in area V5 (estimated from single-unit studies) was covered by TMS. On this latter point, it is probably safe to say that when an experiment deals with sensory functions, a duration of 500 msec from stimulus onset is adequate (see Walsh and Rushworth, 1999).

However, it is not always necessary to identify a site with fMRI. A number of studies have shown clearly that stimulation of the occipital lobe approximately 3 cm dorsal and 5 cm lateral to the inion impairs a range of motion-detection and motion-discrimination tasks and that if the aim of the experiment is to obtain a functional dissociation between motion and some

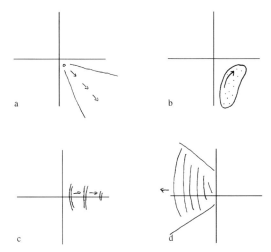

Figure 4.4   Four subjects' impressions of phosphenes elicited by stimulation of area V5. (*a*) The subject described this impression as "movement of a single point in a static field." Stimulation site: left hemisphere 2 cm dorsal and 6 cm lateral to inion; stimulation rate 5 Hz at 1.4 Tesla for 0.5 sec. (*b*) Described as "similar to a random dot array; black dots on a white background; appears to move upwards and rightwards." Stimulation site: left hemisphere 2 cm dorsal and 6 cm lateral to inion; stimulation rate 5 Hz at 1.8 Tesla for 0.5 sec. (*c*) Described as "drifting right, not continuous." Stimulation site: right hemisphere 2 cm dorsal and 5 cm lateral to inion; stimulation rate 10 Hz at 1.4 Tesla for 1 sec. (*d*) Described as "a block of visual noise that jumps to the left." Stimulation site: right hemisphere 2 cm dorsal and 4 cm lateral to inion; stimulation rate single pulse at 1.4 Tesla. The axial bars represent approximately 4 degrees of visual angle. (From Stewart et al., 1999, with permission.)

other visual attribute, such as color, it is sufficient to define the stimulation area functionally rather than anatomically.

Stewart et al. (1999) used the production of moving visual phosphenes to define functionally the location of the movement-specific visual cortex (figure 4.4). Subjects received rTMS at 10 Hz for 0.5 sec and were asked if they saw anything and if what they saw had a shape, color, or direction of movement (a standard procedure for phosphene generation; see Kammer, 1999; Stewart, Walsh, and Rothwell, 2001). When subjects reported movement at a site, this was

assumed to be selectively stimulating the motion area. To corroborate this designation, the production of moving phosphenes was followed by another calibration experiment in which the same area was stimulated to selectively shorten the
duration of the motion aftereffect (figure 4.5) induced by an expanding and ro-
tating field of dots. The level of stimulation was then systematically varied to
establish a phosphene threshold that can be used as an analogue of the motor
threshold. Here, then, is a nonanatomical designation of a stimulation site, which
nevertheless produces similar effects to the sites identified by other means. Following localization of the site, Stewart et al. used rTMS at 10 Hz for 0.5 sec at
80% of phosphene threshold to try to improve learning in a motion task and at
3 Hz for 0.5 sec to try to impair learning on the same task (see chapter 6). The
stimulation parameters were chosen on the basis of a study on visuomotor learning (Pascual-Leone, Bartres-Faz, and Keenan, 1999) with visual phosphene
threshold used in place of motor threshold. Because visual phosphene threshold
and motor thresholds are not correlated (Stewart et al., 2001), it is suggested that
the visual measure be used in vision experiments where possible. It is worth not-
ing that the intensity used in this experiment (80% of phosphene threshold) represents approximately 50% of the stimulator output (MagStim 200 super-rapid
in the labs concerned) and that this intensity is lower than in other studies that
have used V5 stimulation to disrupt motion processing (Hotson et al., 1994;
Beckers and Zeki, 1995; Walsh et al., 1998; Hotson and Anand, 1999; Pascual-
Leone, Bartres-Faz, and Keenan, 1999).

Phosphene thresholds have been found to be stable over time, but
Boroojerdi et al. (2000a, 2000b) have suggested two factors that can change
subjects' sensitivity to stimulation of the occipital cortex. Light deprivation over
a period of 45 min was found to decrease phosphene thresholds by a mean of approximately 12%, and this increase in sensitivity continued until phosphene
thresholds were reduced by approximately 25% from baseline after 3 hr of light
deprivation. After 90 min of deprivation, phosphene thresholds did not return to
baseline for 120 min. On the basis of this experiment, it may be wise to check the
phosphene threshold between blocks of trials during experiments. Repeated

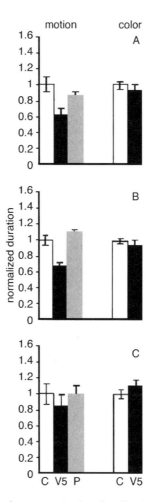

Figure 4.5   Mean duration of motion and color aftereffect in three subjects. C = no TMS.
V5 = TMS over V5, P = TMS over parietal cortex at 10 Hz for 1 sec at the onset of stationary
dots, which previously had been moving for 1 min. Data are normalized to the duration of the
aftereffect with no TMS. (From Stewart et al., 1999, with permission.)

stimulation of the cortex also can change sensitivity, and Boroojerdi et al. noted an increase in phosphene thresholds following 1 Hz stimulation at 100% of baseline threshold for 15 min. However, the increase in thresholds, though statistically significant, was slight (3%), and given the long intertrial intervals in psychological experiments, repeated stimulation is unlikely to change sensitivity sufficiently to influence results where suprathreshold visual stimuli are presented on computer monitors. The same cannot be said for motor deprivation. Temporary restriction or immobilization of limbs can lead to an increase in motor-evoked potentials (MEP) amplitude and an increase in the cortical area from which an MEP can be elicited (Liepert, Teggenthoff, and Malin, 1995; Zanette et al., 1997).

Once lower limits have been set in the literature, it is both advisable and desirable to follow them for scientific as well as ethical reasons. It is more convincing to see an effect of TMS at lower intensities because use of lower intensities reduces the probability that the effect is due to current spread or to other nonspecific variables. It also leads to better control experiments because the location of the control sites, necessary to show specificity, can be closer to the effective site. The control condition need not always be stimulation at a noneffective site; it can be a task control where this is appropriate (see Walsh and Rushworth, 1999). For example, Walsh et al. (1998b) stimulated V5 to produce deficits in tasks requiring complex motion processing, whereas the control tasks demanded complex color and form analysis or simple motion detection. Task controls are used often in single case studies of patients and, of course, are the basis of many neuroimaging experiments.

Most studies using single- or repetitive-pulse TMS apply TMS unilaterally at a single point, but Hotson and colleagues (Hotson et al., 1994; Hotson and Anand, 1999) progressed to simultaneous bilateral stimulation in a study of motion perception. In the first study, TMS was applied unilaterally over the temporo-parieto-occipital junction (TPO) between 50 and 250 msec after the offset of a visual motion display, thus providing a control for the small eye movements they believed may affect results when this region is being stimulated. The effect was to diminish accuracy severely in a random-dot motion task while relatively sparing acuity functions. In the second experiment, TMS was applied at 100% stimulator output intensity (approximately 2.2 Tesla) to each hemisphere. The effect again was to reduce accuracy of motion discrimination and of form-from-motion processing, but this time there was an additional though slight effect on form-from-color detection. The caution here is to wonder about current spread with such high intensities and double-coil stimulation. Even so, what is perhaps notable is that the effect on color processing is rather small. The large intensities used also suggest an explanation for a difference between Hotson et al.'s studies, which observed bilateral visual field motion deficits, and a later study in which the deficits were unilateral but in which the stimulus intensity was lower (Beckers and Zeki, 1995). If effects are obtainable with lower intensities, they are likely to be more specific in terms of range of stimulus types or behaviors affected or the visuotopic spread of deficits. However, Hotson et al.'s observation of unilateral TMS leading to deficits in both visual hemifields has been seen in other studies (Walsh, Ashbridge, and Cowey, 1998), and such deficits may be a behavioral expression of the transcallosal activation reported by Ilmoniemi et al. (1997; see chapter 3). It seems increasingly likely, however, that in a task requiring global motion processing or multiple comparisons of motion in spatially segregated regions of the visual field(s), TMS disruption of any part of the field will be sufficient to degrade performance (cf. Stewart et al., 1999; Campana, Cowey, and Walsh, 2002). Deficits limited to a visual hemifield or even to a region of a hemifield are more likely when the stimulus presentation is short and near the threshold of detection or where the TMS intensity is low. Perceptual reports of the subjects in Hotson et al.'s report compare well with those of Stewart et al.'s subjects (1999) and add to the suggestion of specificity. Subjects receiving TMS over the TPO variously reported "curved, diagonal or zig-zag motion . . . a blurred glimpse of motion . . . [and] the onset and freezing of motion" when TMS was delivered between 100 and 150 msec after stimulus presentation.

Single-pulse experiments present the problem of how to sample time. Imagine that a task takes the subject a second to perform. With rTMS, stimulation can be applied throughout the second, but to stimulate at single-time points 20 msec apart (a not unreasonable temporal window) would increase the number of trials in the experiment by a factor of fifty. It is necessary, therefore, to have at least some temporal hypothesis when using single-pulse TMS. This hypothesis can come from several sources. Corthout et al. (1999a) began with the latencies of single-unit responses in macaque V1 (e.g., Cowey, 1964; Vogels and Orban, 1990; Maunsell and Gibson, 1992; Nowak et al., 1995) and consequently established a functional role for the small population of cells that respond as early as 20 msec after presentation of a visual stimulus. Ashbridge, Walsh, and Cowey (1997) adopted a combination of ERP studies and pilot experiments to investigate visual search and as a result sampled in 20 msec time bins across 200 msec of a task that took approximately 1,000 msec to perform. Evoked potentials were also the source of the stimulation times selected by Zangaladze et al. (1999) in a study of tactile perception, but here TMS was applied only three times after stimulus onset, the intention being to stimulate at one critical time and a control time much as one might stimulate at one critical cortical site and a control site. A similar approach was take by Ganis et al. (2000), who used two TMS stimulation times, based on MEG data in a study of mental rotation. Selection of a small number of stimulation times rather than a temporal window needs careful consideration. As discussed previously, there is reason to believe that TMS interference times may precede ERP peaks. Thus, an apparent unity of critical TMS times and ERP peaks does not mean that the single critical time of an area's contribution to a task has been identified.

A similar train of decisions is seen in motor experiments, but here MRI is rarely used to confirm the locus of stimulation because of the high level of accuracy and reproducibility of the EMG. Motor thresholds typically are set by recording activity elicited from an intrinsic hand muscle such as the abductor pollicis brevis (APB) by TMS over the motor cortex, and threshold is set arbitrarily as the lowest level of stimulation capable of eliciting MEPs of at least 50 μv peak-to-peak amplitude in half of the trials (Wasserman et al., 1992; Wasserman, Pascual-Leone, and Hallett, 1994; Krings et al., 1997; Rossini and Rossi, 1998).

Intrinsic hand muscles are preferred to forearm or upper-arm muscles because their control is almost completely cortical, with minimal spinal contribution (Porter and Lemon, 1993). Stimulation at the threshold site can be used to assess the simple reaction time of a voluntary movement (Day et al., 1989a,b), the time at which a motor command is executed (Schluter et al., 1998), or the involvement of motor cortex in "higher" mental functions (Ganis et al., 2000). In studies of behavior and cognition, the motor threshold has a number of uses. As we saw earlier, in the absence of phosphenes, motor threshold has been used to set the level of stimulation in visual experiments, and, of course, it is used in the same way in motor experiments. Stimulation is expressed as a percentage of motor threshold, which makes it easy to ensure that safety guidelines are being observed (Wassermann, 1998).

More is known about the effects of TMS in the motor system than in the visual system. Applying pulses at low rates of stimulation, say 1 Hz or less, for several minutes can lead to a decrease in cortical excitability (Chen et al., 1997a; Rossi et al., 2000), whereas repeated and sustained TMS at 5 Hz (Berardelli et al., 1998) or higher (Pascual-Leone et al., 1994c) can increase excitability. Thus, any experiment using rTMS should take account of possible changes in the sensitivity of the cortex during a task. A simple precaution that satisfies ethical and scientific concerns is to ensure that intertrain intervals are kept relatively long (5–6 sec or more) to prevent these changes. It is also a good precautionary measure not to use the same subjects on successive days when delivering long trains of rTMS because of wide variations in individual responses to successive days of stimulation (Maeda et al., 2000). These continuing effects of rTMS long beyond the actual time of stimulation can be used to experimental advantage. Kosslyn et al. (1999), for example, applied rTMS at 1 Hz, 90% of motor threshold for 10 min in order to reduce activity in the visual cortex during a later presented visual imagery task. The different effects of high and low rates of rTMS also have been used to probe the role of different motor areas in visuomotor association learning (Pascual-Leone et al., 1999). The effects of low rates of stimulation (1–3 Hz) are found to be robust in these studies, but there is no emerging confidence in the replicability of the effects of higher rates of stimulation, which seem to have different effects not just between studies, but even between different cortical areas (Pascual-Leone et al., 1999; O'Breathnach and Walsh, 1999).

The sampling of time in motor studies is subject to all the points raised in the discussion of the visual system given previously, but there is an additional innovation in motor studies that has not received sufficient attention in the motor field, nor has it transferred to studies of the visual system. Both Day et al. (1989a,b) and Priori et al. (1993) applied single-pulse TMS at a limited number of time points selected on the basis of the subject's known reaction time in the task being carried out. To use this procedure demands temporal knowledge of the task and is thus likely to be more reliable than referring to other ERP or MEG studies made with different subjects and stimulus parameters. It is a method that might prove useful, and reaction-time data from other experiments suggest that it should be a robust means of obtaining behavioral effects (e.g., Ashbridge, Walsh, and Cowey, 1997). It is also another way of thinking of how to narrow the temporal window of single-pulse TMS times. If the experiment is driven by a hypothesis about perceptual aspects of a task, then yoking stimulation to the onset of the sensory stimulus may be the right choice, whereas if the experiment is driven by hypotheses about response components, it may be better to adopt the strategy used by Day et al. and Priori et al. Too few experiments have been carried out to compare these two methods directly to enable one to say categorically which method is best.

SILENT PERIODS AND PAIRED-PULSE PARADIGMS

A single pulse of TMS that evokes a compound motor-action potential on EMG may be followed by a period of significantly decreased electrophysiological activity in the muscle previously activated. This decrease in activity is greatest soon after the MEP is recorded and gradually returns to prepulse levels of baseline activity, sometimes with an overshoot. The length and depth of this silent period depends on several factors, including motor task (Mathis, Quervain, and Hess, 1998), muscle contraction, and stimulus intensity (Triggs et al., 1993).

There is some debate about precisely when the silent period begins and how one should measure it (see Mills, 1999), but the important point here is how it has been used. First, in motor studies, it can be used as a marker of cortical modulation, and thus changes in length or depth due to learning or disease serve as indicators of the site of damage and pathophysiology. Second, because the silent period is independent of previous muscle activity and can be elicited at lower levels of stimulation than MEPs, it is sometimes a more sensitive measure of TMS effects than are MEPs. These factors have been very useful in physiological studies (see Ziemann and Hallet, 2000), but with the exception of plasticity (discussed later) they have not been applied in studies of psychological functions.

A second technique has proven useful to physiologists and does have clear applications in sensory and cognitive studies: The paired-pulse paradigm (Claus et al., 1992; Valls-Solé et al., 1992; Kujirai et al., 1993) measures the effects of a TMS pulse on the EMG responses to a second pulse. The effect of the first pulse depends on its intensity, the interpulse interval, and the intensity of the second pulse. A few general findings from standard paired-pulse experiments of potential use in cognitive studies can be stated. In the standard paradigm (Kujirai et al., 1993), the first (conditioning) pulse is below motor threshold, and the second (test) pulse is above motor threshold. In that case, short interstimulus intervals (1–5 msec) can produce intracortical inhibition, and slightly longer intervals (7–30 msec) produce facilitation. The mechanisms of these effects have been shown to be mediated by different cortical mechanisms. For example, lower-intensity conditioning pulses are required more for inhibition than for excitation; coil orientation and thus direction of current flow are critical for excitation but not inhibition; and the two phenomena can be affected independently by drugs and neurological disease. Paired-pulse paradigms have only begun to be introduced to psychological studies (Oliveri et al., 2000), but the ability to increase or decrease sensitivity of a cortical region over a short period of time has clear applications awaiting it in studies of priming, threshold detection, and cortical interactions.

SITES OF STIMULATION

Glory to your imperfections.

—*Pedro Salinas*

Motor cortex in particular and visual cortex to a lesser extent may be considered the "easy meat" of TMS because there are tell-tale signs—MEPs and phosphenes—of where one is stimulating. For the cognitive neuroscientist, however, the brain regions of interest are often likely to be one of Penfield and Rasmussen's "elaboration areas,"[2] which do not have reliable stimulation signatures such as phosphenes or MEPs. Even so it is not always necessary to use MRI as the means of localization; indeed, even if one does so, one will still have to establish a behavioral effect. Imagine a single-unit physiologist advancing his electrode. The physiologist hunts for the desired response and then works on the specificity of the cell. The behavior in a TMS experiment can be similar. Ashbridge, Walsh, and Cowey (1997) introduced a "hunting paradigm" for TMS in the elaboration areas. A site for the application of TMS is selected on the basis of previous studies that have published scalp coordinates or that include reference to ERP electrode sites that may be relevant. That site is then marked on the subject's head and forms the center of a grid of points marked 1 cm apart. To stimulate all points at all single-pulse intervals would give rise to the same combinatorial explosion of trials caused by not having a temporal hypothesis, and subjects also may be learning the task as the experimenter spends several hundred trials failing to get any effects. There are three and one-half solutions to this problem. Following pilot experiments or physiological data as discussed earlier, a researcher can select one or two stimulus-onset asynchrony times and sample all the points for ten to twenty trials until an effective site is found. Using rTMS

---

2. Elaboration areas are regions from which no overt response was elicited by direct electrical stimulation by Penfield and colleagues. They said of these areas that stimulation "sheds no light upon the function of an area unless the patient is making use of that area at the moment" (Penfield and Rasmussen, 1950, 234).

is more effective, and the site found to produce a behavioral effect then can be used in a follow-up single-pulse experiment. The third way is to use a behavioral assay. One example is the use of visual search tasks to identify the posterior parietal cortex (PPC). Rushworth, Ellison, and Walsh (2001) applied rTMS over several sites around coordinates at which TMS had been shown to disrupt visual search (Ashbridge, Walsh, and Cowey, 1997). When a disrupted search was noted, measured by an increase in reaction times, the effective site then was used in an experiment to disrupt visual orienting. As more data accrue on the effects of TMS on cognition, it will become easier to rely on such behavioral assays. The half solution to the problem of site location is to use a site such as the motor cortex as a reference point from which to measure along the scalp to, say, premotor cortex (Schluter et al., 1998), frontal eye fields (Muri, Hess, and Meienberg, 1991; Muri, Rosler, and Hess, 1994; Muri et al., 1995, 1996, 1999; Ro et al., 1999), or Broca's area (Pascual-Leone et al., 1993c). This is only a partial solution because of intersubject variability in the relative location of cortical areas, and the hunting paradigm therefore would need to be employed again and possibly over an undesirably large area. Using the hunting method with small numbers of trials runs the risk of false negatives—sites being rejected—when more trials may yield an effect. This is an occupational hazard that has to be faced by experimental judgment. It is not unique to TMS (cf. debates on false positive in fMRI studies).

Perhaps Hubel, who experienced the problem of sampling bias in single-unit studies, can help here. Hubel and Wiesel, in their studies on orientation columns in V1, did not note the preponderance of chromatic responsive cells with poor orientation selectivity in laminae 2 and 3. In later years, Hubel recorded extensively from these cells and commented,

> The historically minded reader may have wondered how so prominent a group of cells could have been missed by so prominent a pair of investigators (e.g. Hubel and Wiesel, 1968). We, of course, wondered the same thing and can think of several possible reasons. (1) Injured cells become sensitive to almost any visual stimulus so that orientation selectivity can be lowered or lost. Thus lack of

orientation was probably sometimes wrongly imputed to injury. (2) With no anatomical indication of non-homogeneity in the upper cortical layers, it would have been easy to dismiss occasional, apparently sporadic groups of unoriented cells. (3) A sudden series of monocular non-oriented cells could be interpreted as entering Layer 4C, which occasionally might have seemed remarkably superficial. (4) The prominence was ill-begotten (Livingstone and Hubel, 1984).

Glory to those imperfections indeed.

LESS IS . . . WELL, JUST LESS SOMETIMES

Before researchers embark on a single-pulse study with the intention of testing a hypothesis about the critical timing of an area's involvement in a task, it may be worthwhile for them to establish that an effect can be produced with rTMS. However, the fact that rTMS can produce deficits is no guarantee that single-pulse TMS also will produce deficits. Prior to the demonstrations of single-pulse TMS effects on visual search (Ashbridge, Walsh, and Cowey, 1997), cognitive tasks required rTMS to produce effects, which may not be because of any deficiencies in the attempts to disrupt cognition, but rather because some functions are relatively redundant with respect to time and therefore lack the sequential processing necessary to allow single-pulse TMS to create sufficient neural noise to disrupt the task. It seems that the more anterior one travels in the cortex, away from sensory and motor areas, the more likely it is that functions require rTMS to produce disruptions. Two exceptions to this rule (Haggard and Magno, 1999; Schluter et al., 1998; see chapter 5) used task designs in which the sequence of information-processing stages was explicit and also used reaction time as the dependent variable, but other tasks or functions may be more difficult to break down. Speech production, for example, which so far has been disrupted only with rTMS, requires a cascade of interactions between areas in the frontal lobe that are responsible for selecting words and generating motor programs and the motor areas responsible for direct output to the facial muscles. The critical elements here are feedback and task complexity. Speech disruptions with stimulation of the motor cortex cannot be achieved by single-pulse TMS, but this does not mean that speech and language functions cannot be studied using single-pulse TMS as long as the apparently complex task is broken down into components amenable to interference. Again, a reaction time or deadline paradigm seems to offer the best possibilities, and studies of the many areas involved in the different stages of language perception and production are already emerging (e.g., Stewart et al., 2000).

FACILITATIONS: BEWARE OF FALSE PROFITS

One of the most intriguing effects of TMS is the enhancement of performance in some way—usually the speed of response. Where this is a genuine and specific improvement of function, it can lead to new insights about cortical functions. However, one's first response to improvements caused by TMS should be caution because there is good evidence that TMS can decrease reaction times— nonspecifically to auditory, visual, or somatosensory stimuli (Pascual-Leone et al., 1992a, 1992b)—by mechanisms related to intersensory facilitation (Terao et al., 1998a,b).

TMS might speed up reaction time by subthreshold stimulation of the motor representation of the responding hand when simple motor responses are required to "go" signals. However, such an effect might represent nonspecific reaction-time decreases that have to be ruled out carefully. For example, the simple decision of whether to block TMS trials or interleave them with non-TMS trials depends on the duration of stimulus presentation, the type of TMS (single or repetitive pulse), the duration of the train, and the kind of response required. Take the following scenario: The stimulus is presented for 500 msec; single-pulse TMS is applied at either 100, 250, or 500 msec after stimulus onset; and the response required is a finger press for reaction-time measurement. Subjects easily can perceive the difference between 100, 250, and 500 msec, and one consequence may be that in blocks of trials in which TMS is delivered on every trial, subjects simply wait, albeit unwittingly, for TMS to be delivered before making

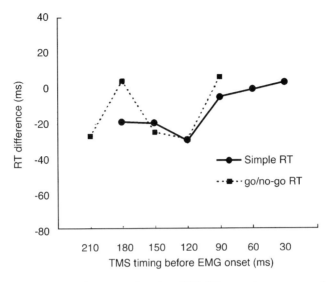

Figure 4.6   Comparison of mean reaction-time (RT) differences between control trials and trials on which TMS is applied to the motor cortex contralateral to the hand of response in a simple choice reaction-time task (circles and solid line) and a go/no-go task (squares, dotted line). (From Sawaki et al., 1999, with permission.)

their response, leaving the experimenter with long reaction times, no less than 500 msec in this case. If TMS is delivered on random trials, then the experimenter runs the risk of alerting the subjects and obtaining artifactually fast reaction times. Some piloting of the best kind of arrangement is necessary in all behavioral experiments, and the results may influence the type of experiment designed. Sawaki et al. (1999), for example, showed that reaction-time decreases could be obtained either early (0 msec stimulus-TMS delay) in a simple reaction-time task and in a "go/no go" task requiring thumb abduction or later in the task when TMS was applied 90 msec after presentation of the "go" signal in the conditional task but not in the simple reaction-time task. Figure 4.6 shows the difference between the two effects—the early effect could be elicited by stimulation of the contralateral motor cortex or over parietal electrode site P4, whereas the later effect could be elicited only with TMS over the contralateral motor cortex. Sawaki et al. concluded that the early effect in simple reaction-time tasks is due to intersensory facilitation and that the later effect is more likely due to motor-specific variables. Even so, stimulation at control sites may yield reaction-time changes due to the subject's state of anticipation or surprise at the delivery of the pulse. One elegant solution to speeding of responses can be seen in an experiment by Marzi and colleagues (1998). In this experiment, subjects were required to make manual responses to a visual stimulus presented to the same (uncrossed condition) or different (crossed condition) cerebral hemisphere as the responding hand (figure 4.7). Figure 4.8 shows the results. Note that the acoustic click of the stimulator had an equal facilitatory effect on crossed and uncrossed trials. Note also that the TMS facilitatory effect on the re-action time in the crossed condition (visual stimulus presented to the hemi-sphere ipsilateral to the responding hand) was smaller than in the uncrossed condition. Marzi and colleagues interpreted this *difference* between the facilita-tions as the deficit caused by TMS. This kind of analysis shares the logic of sub-traction used in fMRI studies and, of course, demands a detailed understanding of the task being used. Flitman et al. (1998) used a similar approach to analysis in the study of linguistic processing (see "Lost for Words," chapter 6).

Subjects, intersensory facilitation, motor facilitation, subtractions of acoustic artifacts, and task-dependent causes of enhancements are some of things a researcher should bear in mind when presented with unexpected enhance-ments. Anatomy, neuropsychology, brain-imaging data, and speed-accuracy trade-offs are also important. In cognitive tasks, reaction times can be a more sensitive and robust measure than errors because errors are so difficult to produce with suprathreshold stimuli, but an analysis of changes in accuracy as a function of changes in speed may reveal that what appears to be an improvement in reaction time is bought at the expense of making more errors in the task. If the enhancement obtained is task specific, then it is worth considering whether magnetic stimulation of an area may decrease the inhibitory effect that area has on anatomically connected neighbors. For example, Seyal, Ro, and Rafal (1995) obtained decreases in tactile thresholds in the fingers ipsilateral to the hemi-sphere of stimulation in the somatosensory cortex, but their data can be

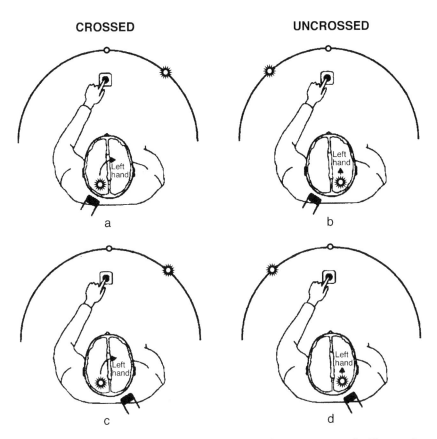

Figure 4.7 Interhemispheric visuomotor interaction. Subjects are presented with a cue in one of the two visual fields and required to respond with right or left hand (left hand only shown here). In the crossed-hemisphere condition, hemifield and hand are represented in opposite hemispheres (*a* and *c*), and in the uncrossed condition they are represented in the same hemisphere (*b* and *d*). TMS was applied to the responding or stimulated hemisphere. (From Marzi et al., 1998, with permission.)

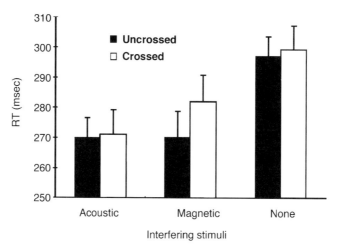

Figure 4.8   Reaction times for the crossed and uncrossed conditions for three types of TMS interference. There was a general facilitatory effect of TMS, caused by intersensory facilitation due to the acoustic click. TMS also had a specific effect in delaying the crossed reaction times relative to the uncrossed. (From Marzi et al., 1998, with permission.)

explained on the basis of diminished competition between the two hemispheres. The task-specific enhancements reported by Walsh et al. (1998), wherein TMS over visual area V5 enhanced performance on color/form conjunction tasks, are due to release of areas involved in color and form perception (presumably areas V4 and TEO) from competition with V5. Both Seyal, Ro, and Rafal's and Walsh et al.'s studies carried strong predictions based on anatomical connections, and neither contradicted the direction of effects seen in neuropsychological patients. If the enhancements seen do flatly contradict neuropsychological data—for example, if TMS over V5 had led to an improvement in performance on motion tasks—then one would have to have strong a priori expectations to be able to begin to justify them. In experiments where the aim is to disrupt a specific task, TMS is likely to be applied at an intensity well above motor or phosphene threshold; thus, it is rare to see selective enhancements on the task that one is aiming to disrupt.

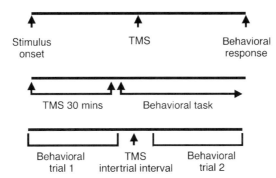

Figure 4.9   Different temporal modes of disruptive TMS. Magnetic stimulation can be applied after the onset of some imperative signal or discriminanda in order to produce a slowing of or errors in the response (*top*). The stimulation can be single, double, or repetitive pulse. In the distal method (*middle*), TMS is applied for several minutes before the subject performs a task. The stimulation in this method is always repetitive, usually 1–3 Hz to decrease activity in the areas stimulated. An intermediate mode (*bottom*) is to use TMS between the trials of a perceptual or cognitive task to disrupt processing that may consolidate events of the previous trial or preparatory processes for the upcoming trial.

TUNING IN AND TURNING OFF

The importance of correct interpretation of enhancements extends to a completely different type of study in which rTMS can be used to change the excitability of cortex over a period of several minutes beyond the application of the cortical stimulation. Here the experimenter runs into one of the problems we have been arguing TMS can meet—namely, cortical reorganization—and also the difficulties mentioned previously regarding the variable effects of high-frequency rTMS. If the effects of rTMS are to be understood in full, it is important to be able to correlate the physiological product of stimulation with behavioral consequences. The class of experiments this correlation requires is different from the type we have discussed so far. The three experimental time lines in figure 4.9 show how the paradigms differ. In one paradigm, TMS is applied *during* the performance of the task, and it is a simple matter of parsimony to interpret the effects of TMS as being due to neural noise. In the second paradigm, TMS is applied for several minutes *before* the subject is tested on the task of interest, and the effects of TMS are interpreted as due to the residual physiological changes caused by the stimulation. In the third paradigm, introduced by Campana, Cowey, and Walsh (2002), TMS is used in an intermediate manner by applying pulses during a block of trials but doing so in the intertrial period rather than before a block of trials (distal method) or during task performance (normal interference mode). This method can be used to test hypotheses about consolidation of events, priming, or short-term memory (see "Perceptual Memory: A New Window for TMS and Psychophysics," chapter 6).

To investigate changes in cortical excitability caused by TMS in the second paradigm shown in figure 4.9 (the distal paradigm), Chen et al. (1997a) applied 0.1 Hz TMS to the motor cortex and observed elevations in evoked motor threshold as a result. Wang and colleagues (Wang, Wang, and Scheich, 1996; Wang et al., 1999) observed similar effects, indicative of long-term depression in the auditory behavior of gerbils and have pursued the effects of distal TMS by assessing changes in evoked activity following long trains of rTMS and by seeking to correlate the physiological effects with the consequences for behavior. Gerbils were given rTMS (5 Hz; 3 Tesla; 5 min to 1 sec on, 5 secs off, until the animals had received 250 pulses) on four sessions a day, and each TMS session was followed by training on an auditory discrimination task. Other animals received rTMS and underwent electrophysiological stimulation and recording for up to 24 hr following TMS. The electrophysiological study showed that a single rate of rTMS could evoke an increase in long-term depression that lasted up to 24 hr or in long-term potentiation that lasted up to 3 hr. No reason for the induction of long-term depression or potentiation in different trials and animals was obvious other than the system's intrinsic variability. The effect of TMS on behavior was to slow down the rate of learning. Studies that have attempted to enhance and inhibit cortical activity selectively in human cortex present a slightly more consistent but no less paradoxical picture.

One area of agreement seems to be that low-frequency rTMS decreases cortical excitability both during (Pascual-Leone et al., 1994c; Jennum, Winkel, and Fuglsang-Frederiksen, 1995) and following stimulation (Chen et al., 1997a; Tergau et al., 1997; Pascual-Leone et al., 1998b). An area of less agreement is that stimulation at 5 Hz or 10 Hz unambiguously increases excitability. Maeda et al. (2000) applied rTMS at 1, 10, or 20 Hz over a two-day period and measured changes in motor thresholds. Elevations in MEP thresholds were observed on both days with 1 Hz TMS, and decreases in threshold were obtained following 20 Hz stimulation, but there were no effects from 10 Hz stimulation. As Maeda et al. emphasize, however, the individual variability in these subjects was large, and the reproducibility of effects was low. Part of the problem here lies in the variability of the persistence of TMS effects. If subjects show marked differences in motor threshold, one might as reasonably expect their cortical systems to show variability in the rate of recovery from stimulation. Studies variously have obtained changes in cortical activity ranging from 3 to 4 min (Pascual-Leone et al., 1994) to 10 min (Fox et al., 1997). The only safe conclusion one can draw at this point in time is that changes in cortical activity as a result of distal rTMS can vary in direction and duration as a function of stimulation frequency, intensity, intertrain interval, train duration, and the total number of pulses. This is not a matter for despair, but for investigation. There is yet another caveat, however. The effects of distal rTMS may differ also as a function of the area to be stimulated for a given task. For example, Pascual-Leone et al. (1999b) applied 1 Hz and 10 Hz TMS to either the motor cortex or dorsolateral prefrontal cortex of subjects performing an implicit visuomotor learning task. As figure 4.10 shows, 10 Hz stimulation over the motor cortex led to an increase in the rate at which the subjects acquired the association, whereas the same stimulation over the dorsolateral prefrontal cortex impeded learning. To interpret effects such as these, one needs to understand not only the effects of frequency, intensity, duration, and so on, but also a good deal about the role of the cortical area under investigation in the task presented to the subjects.

Distal rTMS can be used to test specific predictions regarding cortical function, and if we were to offer a methodological heuristic here, it would be to keep the task as simple as possible and preferably limited to stimuli about which a great deal of physiology is known. This means that distal rTMS is likely to be

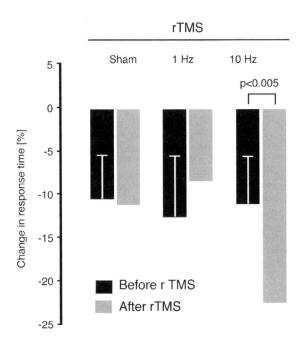

Figure 4.10 The effect of modulation of excitability of motor cortex by rTMS on procedural learning in a serial reaction-time task. Subjects received either sham, 1 Hz, or 10 Hz TMS. The 10 Hz TMS clearly reduced the reaction time—that is, improved performance.

most successful when used in primary or sensory areas where the body of physiological knowledge can provide a brake on the possible interpretations of results. Taking this approach and going along with the emerging consensus that low-frequency TMS tends to have inhibitory consequences on cortical activity, Kosslyn et al. (1999) used 1 Hz stimulation to test the hypothesis that the primary visual cortex is important in visual imagery (see "Necessity and Efficiency," chapter 6), and Stewart et al. (1999) employed the same rationale in an attempt to reduce learning in a visual motion-discrimination task with 3 Hz stimulation over V5 (see "Perceptual Learning," chapter 6).

THE FUTURE OF VIRTUAL PATIENTS

In this chapter, we have provided a warts-and-all account of the creation of virtual patients. We have done so because the warts will be easy to remove as understanding of the effects of TMS increases. There are indeed several factors that constrain the choice of task, dependent variable, locus of stimulation, direction of effects, and interpretation of results, but these constraints underlie the value of TMS; the caution they encourage is welcome. The most parsimonious account of the effects of TMS in cognitive tasks is at present the neural noise account, and it should be extended to interpretation of the effects of distal rTMS, especially where performance enhancement is obtained. If rTMS makes a subject better at a task, the mechanism is more likely to be that TMS introduced neural noise into an inhibitory component of the processing rather than enhanced the organized activity of the processes that contribute directly to the output of the task.

The kinds of virtual patients one can produce fall into the four categories shown in figure 4.11. TMS can be used to produce errors or deficits by disrupting the primary function of focus either on-line or distally (figure 4.11, top) or by inducing neural noise at a secondary site (figure 4.11), the effect of which may be to disinhibit function in a second area (figure 4.11), which may lead to a paradoxical improvement in the task. Double virtual lesions also can be used to assess interactions between areas (figure 4.11, bottom), or distal rTMS can be given to induce a primary virtual lesion, to which a second single-pulse virtual lesion can be added as a way of investigating necessary interactions between areas. The type of "lesion" one wants to induce depends on the question being asked: The difference with TMS, vis-à-vis classical neuropsychology, is that one can now select the lesion for the question rather than select questions determined by the availability of the lesion.

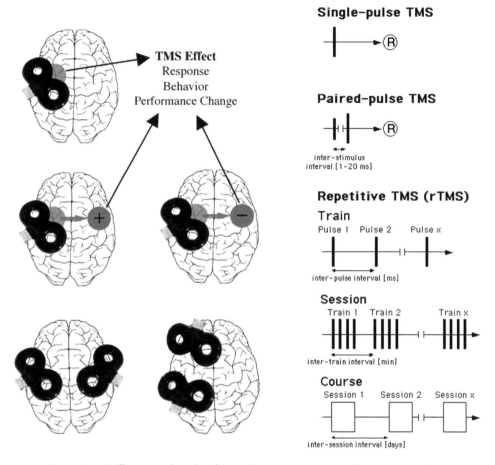

Figure 4.11   Different spatial modes of TMS. The most common use of magnetic stimulation is to apply pulses over a single brain area of interest to influence the area under the coil directly (*first panel*). TMS also can disrupt activity at a secondary site, the effects of which may be positive (*second panel*) or negative (*third panel*) depending on the functions of the areas connected. TMS also can be applied to two sites simultaneously or with some given stimulation-onset asynchrony to investigate the timing of the interactions of two areas (e.g., Pascual-Leone and Walsh, 2001; *bottom panel*).

REAL-TIME NEUROPSYCHOLOGY: SINGLE-PULSE TMS

WHAT'S WRONG WITH NEUROPSYCHOLOGY? NOTHING, BUT . . .

Neuropsychological studies of patients provide one of the cornerstones upon which much of our knowledge of the neurological basis of cognition is built. Another one of those cornerstones is the wealth of data and models produced by more than a century of experimental psychology. There is a yawning gap between these two bodies of knowledge, however. Consider what they offer. Studies of patients rely on dissociable effects of brain damage (Shallice, 1988). One example, to which we return later in this chapter and again in chapter 6, is the difference between the effects of damage to the left and right parietal cortices. Patients with right parietal damage can have deficits in visual search and eye movements or neglect of the contralateral side of space. Left-hemisphere damage, however, rarely produces visual problems but is more likely to lead to deficits that appear to be motor homologues of right-hemisphere damage—for example, intention deficits (Rushworth, Ellison, and Walsh, 2001). It would be a caricature of classical neuropsychology to say that it has delivered information only about *where* in the brain a function might be performed. It in fact has given us a body of functional knowledge about how component functions might be organized in the brain. It is not unfair to say, however, that neuropsychological studies cannot deal with the dynamic, real-time interactions between cortical areas. Patients are often slow to perform tasks, and it is common to find that a task that can be run as a reaction-time study in normal subjects can only be run using errors as the dependent variable in patients. In other words, studies of neuropsychological patients have poor temporal resolution.

On the other hand, experimental psychology and psychophysics are replete with temporal resolution. Shepard and Metzeler (1971), for example, were able to calculate the speed at which objects can be rotated mentally, and in visual search tasks each additional distracter can be accorded a number of milliseconds to be processed (see, for example, Treisman, 1988, 1996; Duncan and Humphreys, 1989; Wolfe, 1994). These and other psychological models are perhaps the richest source of information and theories about the *when* and *how* of information processing. Just as neuropsychological studies are devoid of temporal resolution, many psychological studies do not address brain function and localization. One of the functions of this book is to describe the contribution the use of TMS can make to bridging the gap between spatial and temporal resolution, between neuropsychological experimental results and psychological models.

In the updated preface to his book *Chronometric Explorations of Mind* (1978, 1986), Posner noted that the general approach to chronometry was enhanced greatly by the use of brain scans and MEG. The work discussed in this book does not change the basic story of chronometric exploration but forms a new chapter in the venture. As we noted in chapter 4, the virtual-patient approach allows one to create deficits limited to time windows of 10 or 20 msec, and it is to some of these experiments we now turn to examine the value of single-pulse TMS.

TIMES PAST: THE WATERSHED STUDIES OF VISION AND MOVEMENT

One of the tenets of experimental psychology is that any given stage of information processing takes a finite amount of time. Psychological models reflect both the sequencing of events and, in some cases, the veridical time windows

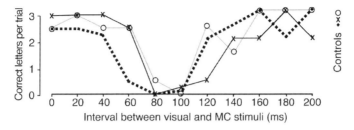

Figure 5.1   Visual suppression curves of three subjects. The proportion of correct identifica-
tions of three dark letters briefly flashed on a bright background is plotted as a function of the
delay between stimulus onset and the application of TMS pulse over the occipital visual cortex. The magnetic stimulation was delivered with a round coil (MC). (From Amassian et al.,
1989, with permission.)

of component processes. A classic example is that of backward visual masking
(Michaels and Turvey, 1979). If two visual stimuli are presented close enough
together in time (the exact time depends on the similarity of the two stimuli
and the duration of presentation), the second stimulus will impede identification of the first. Amassian and colleagues (1989) were the first to use TMS as a
virtual-lesion technique in the visual system[3] and also the first to extend this
technique to probe the cortical basis of the well-established psychological phenomenon of visual masking (Amassian et al., 1993a, 1993b). In the first experiment, subjects were presented with small, low-contrast trigrams and required
to identify the three letters. TMS was applied using a round coil with the lower
edge approximately 2 cm above inion. Pulses were given once per trial at a visual stimulus–TMS onset asynchrony of between 0 and 200 msec. Figure 5.1
shows that TMS was effective in abolishing the subjects' ability to identify the
letter if the pulse was delivered between 80 and 100 msec after onset of the visual stimuli. They also demonstrated the retinotopic specificity of the effect by
moving the coil slightly to the left, causing a decrease in identifying only letters on the right of the trigram, or by moving the coil to the right, causing a

3. The first use of the virtual-lesion technique in the motor system was by Day et al. (1989a,b).
Because of its methodological importance, this experiment is discussed in detail in chapter 4.

corresponding decrease in identifying letters to the left. Finally, they also used vertical trigrams and showed that moving the coil dorsally disrupted perception of the lower letter and that moving it ventrally interrupted reports of the upper letters.

Most experimenters would have been satisfied at having peered through a relatively small time window during which visual cortex is critical for letter identification, but Amassian and colleagues were not satisfied with using TMS merely to make subjects worse on a task. To make a real test of the specificity of the technique, they needed to exclude the possibility that TMS had not made subjects worse on the task because of nonspecific effects on vision. To demonstrate that TMS was having specific effects, it should be possible to find an example of two competing stimulus loads and to use TMS to disrupt one selectively in order to unmask the other. Amassian and colleagues used a classical visual-masking paradigm in which subjects were presented with an initial trigram of target letters followed 100 msec later by a second set of masking letters. Following this second set of letters, TMS was applied at a trigram-TMS onset asynchrony of 0 to 200 msec (figure 5.2). The presentation of the second set of letters clearly masks the processing of the first, presumably due to some overlapping time period during which initial processing of the second set prevented access to the results of processing the first set. When TMS was applied over the occipital cortex, however, the effects of the second set of stimuli were removed. TMS masked processing of the second set in order to unmask processing of the first, and the time course of the TMS unmasking effect mirrored that of the original masking effect (figure 5.2).

Amassian's work is a good example of how to fuse TMS with psychological models, and it laid the foundation for other visual TMS studies, but questions remain. For example, occipital pole stimulation may include several visual areas, and other experiments are required to clarify which neural processes correspond with the different psychological components of visual tasks. The optimal latency of the TMS effect on suppression and masking (80–100 msec) led Amassian et al. to suggest that the critical site of stimulation lay beyond the striate cortex. Corthout et al. (1999a,b) disrupted identification of centrally

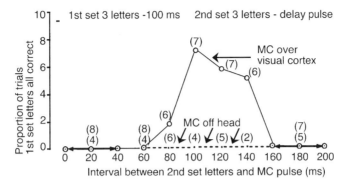

Figure 5.2   Masking of the first trigram produced by the presentation of a second trigram can be unmasked by TMS suppression of the second trigram. The proportion of trials in which the subjects correctly reported all the letters of the first trigram are presented as a function of the delay between the presentation of the second trigram and the TMS pulse. Numbers in parentheses are the number of trials with TMS (*higher row of numbers*) and with sham TMS (*lower row of numbers*). MC, magnetic coil. (From Amassian et al., 1993a, with permission.)

presented letter targets with occipital stimulation as early as 20 msec after stimulus onset, consistent with some reports from single-unit physiology of V1 responses (Wilson et al., 1983; Celebrini et al., 1993; Schmolesky et al., 1998). However, early/late effective stimulation times may not always mean that lower/higher levels of the visual system are being disrupted, and it would not be difficult to launch the counter explanation that late effects of TMS may be due to disruption of back projections to V1 rather than to disruption of extrastriate areas (see Hupe et al., 2001; Pascual-Leone and Walsh, 2001). Equating TMS time with the cortical stage of processing demands corroborating evidence such as supporting single-unit physiology (see Zangaladze et al., 1999) or knowledge of anatomical connections (see Marzi et al., 1998).

Amassian's work was illustrative and elegant and provided the spur for TMS studies to go further and to produce virtual patients who show deficits that will yield new dissociations and generate reassessments of the neuropsychological findings.

RELATIVE TIME: ADDING TO THE NEUROPSYCHOLOGY

Patients with damage to the right parietal cortex may exhibit a range of deficits that include detection of a conjunction target in a visual search array (Arguin, Joanette, and Cavanagh, 1990, 1993; Friedman-Hill, Robertson, and Treisman, 1995), inability to attend to the left side of visual space (Bisiach and Vallar, 1988; Weintraub and Mesulam, 1987; Bisiach et al., 1990, 1994, 1996), and inaccurate saccadic eye movements. The first two deficits often are linked together, and one explanation of these patients' failure to detect conjunction targets is that their spatial attentional problems prevent them from performing what is referred to as "visual binding" (Treisman, 1996). The posterior parietal cortex lies on the dorsolateral surface of the cortex and is easily accessible to TMS. In an attempt to model the effects of right parietal lesions, a number of single-pulse studies have been carried out. Ashbridge, Walsh, and Cowey (1997) stimulated right PPC while subjects carried out standard "feature" and "conjunction" visual search tasks (figure 5.3). Patients with right PPC lesions are impaired on the conjunction tasks but not on the feature tasks. TMS over the right PPC replicated these two basic findings but with some important differences. Single pulses of TMS were applied at stimulus–TMS onset asynchronies of between 0 and 200 msec, and subjects showed two patterns of effect. The reaction time to report "target present" was increased maximally when TMS was applied approximately 100 msec after visual stimulus onset, but to increase the time taken to report "target absent" TMS had to be applied approximately 160 msec after visual array onset (figure 5.4). Here, then, TMS has replicated the patient data (PPC damage impairs conjunction search), but it adds two further items of information—that the PPC is important for "target absent" responses and that the mechanisms underlying "target present" and "target absent" responses occupy different time windows in the PPC. The finding with "target absent" responses is an important addition to the studies of binding deficits in patients with parietal damage (e.g., Friedman-Hill, Robertson, and Treisman, 1995). In those studies, the patients typically make illusory conjunction errors and thus bias interpretation to one

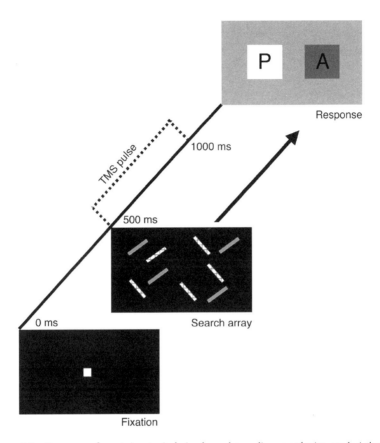

Figure 5.3   Sequence of events in a typical visual search paradigm, employing mode 1 shown in figure 4.11. A fixation spot on the monitor is followed by the array for 500 msec and a single pulse or a repetitive train of TMS is applied at some point in the time window between array onset and responding "present" (P) or "absent" (A).

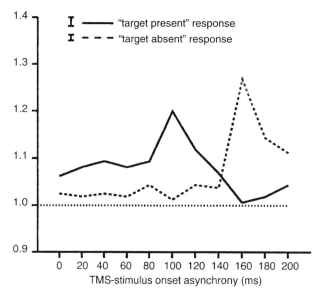

Figure 5.4 The effects of TMS applied over the right PPC of naive subjects on a conjunction visual search task (with eight stimuli in the array). Data are normalized to the reaction time on trials when search was performed without TMS. TMS had a clear effect in trials when the target was present if the pulse was delivered 100 msec after stimulus onset and also when the target was absent if the pulse was delivered 160 msec after target onset. Vertical bars represent ±1 standard error. (From Walsh et al., 1997, with permission.)

based on stimulus-driven processes. The effects on "target absent" trials, however, suggest that response-driven factors need also be considered.

As we noted earlier, patients often have an array of problems, which means that standard psychological experimental paradigms have to be modified, and reaction-time studies might be problematic. In studies of visual search, the patients are likely to report a high level of false positives, and thus we have little knowledge from them about how the PPC might contribute to search in the absence of the target. Indeed, because of the patients' propensity to report positively, the deficit has been interpreted predominantly as one of visual binding. Ashbridge, Walsh, and Cowey's (1997) "target absent" data require that this conclusion be reconsidered. If PPC is important to *both* "target present" and "target absent" trials, it is unlikely that its special role in visual search is binding the separate features of the target—in "target absent" trials there is no target to bind. The answer to the role of PPC lies in the relative timing of the TMS effects on "target present" and "target absent" responses. "Target present" responses typically occur more quickly than "target absent" responses (784 msec and 856 msec, respectively, in the experiment discussed here), and the order of the TMS effects mirror this difference. This result has been observed in many subsequent studies. A parsimonious interpretation of these data is that the PPC contribution is not to the components of search that involve binding of visual attributes, for which the extrastriate visual areas seem sufficient (Corbetta et al., 1991, 1995), but rather to the response component of search (Ellison et al., submitted). Later experiments have reinforced some aspects of this interpretation (see chapter 6).

Conjunction searches used in experiments to compare performance with feature searches usually are selected to yield a serial search function; likewise, the feature searches are selected because they return a flat reaction-time/set size slope. Thus, a parietal cortex–damaged patient's failure to detect conjunction targets accurately may be due to the difficulty of identifying conjunctions relative to features, rather than to anything intrinsic to feature binding. To investigate this problem, Ellison et al. (submitted) gave subjects difficult and easy feature and conjunction search tasks to dissociate the importance of binding from difficulty. The easy feature and conjunction tasks were performed with a flat search function, and the difficult feature and conjunction searches gave a serial function and longer intercepts than the easy tasks. Figure 5.5 shows the four tasks used. TMS was given over the right PPC at 10 Hz for 500 msec at approximately 60% of stimulator output at the onset of the visual array. TMS significantly lengthened reaction times on the two conjunction tasks but had no effect on the two feature tasks. From this experiment, then, it seems that the parietal cortex does have an important role in some element of conjunction searches. In their next experiment, Ellison et al. used the same targets and distractors but presented them as singletons on each trial, and the subject now had to decide whether the stimulus present was a target or a distractor (figure 5.6). In one condition, the stimulus was always presented in the center of the computer monitor,

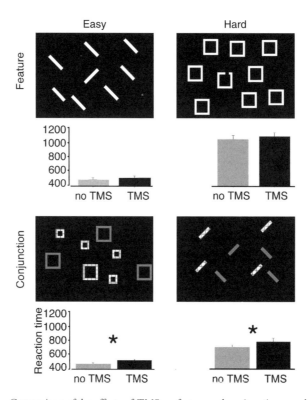

Figure 5.5   Comparison of the effects of TMS on feature and conjunction search tasks independent of whether performance on the task is hard or easy. TMS was applied over the right PPC in seven subjects. TMS caused an increase in reaction times when the visual search array presented the subjects with a conjunction task irrespective of task difficulty. TMS did not have any effect on the performance of feature-discrimination tasks even when the feature task was more difficult (defined as taking longer per item in the display) than a conjunction task that was disrupted by TMS.

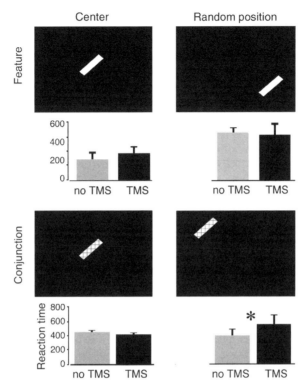

Figure 5.6   The effects of TMS on identifying the presence or absence of a conjunction target are not significant when the spatial location of the discriminanda is known and there are no distractors in the array.

and in the other condition the stimulus could appear anywhere on the monitor. As figure 5.6 shows, TMS over the right PPC did not affect the subjects' reaction time for detection of the conjunction target when it was in the center of the monitor, but it did slow down the subjects when the stimulus could appear anywhere on the screen. The combined results of these two experiments suggest that the PPC is important for conjunction detection but only when the spatial location of the appearance of the stimulus is uncertain. This hypothesis could be taken as consistent with the claim that the PPC is necessary for the spatial processing that is a prerequisite of visual binding (Friedman-Hill, Robertson, and Treisman, 1995). However, the lack of TMS effects on the conjunction-detection task in the center-only condition weakens an account based on binding of features.

A clue to the function of the PPC is in its anatomical location—poised between the visual and motor cortices; it would seem that the critical role of PPC in visual search is visuomotor, perhaps an involvement in initially forming stimulus-response associations. An alternative view of Ellison et al.'s data, therefore, would be to interpret the TMS costs incurred when spatial uncertainty is introduced to the task as a cost in deciding where in space to direct one's response. A third experiment also favors a response-based view rather than a visual-binding account of the PPC function in search. The increase in reaction time remained relatively constant across set sizes and is not related to the number of elements in the visual array. Any function disrupted as a function of a visual component of the task might be expected to be disrupted increasingly as the visual component of the task increased.

The PPC is also important for eye movements, and two types of movement have been investigated with TMS. The benchmark study (Priori et al., 1993) applied single pulses of TMS with a circular coil placed over the vertex. Subjects fixated a point and were required to saccade to it when it jumped 11 degrees either to the right or left of fixation. Following the same methodological rationale as Day et al. (1989b), Priori et al. applied TMS 60 msec before the expected saccade onset time measured by electro-oculogram (EOG). The mean reaction time was increased from 189 msec by 40 to 50 msec although amplitude and duration were unaffected. This is again consistent with the neural noise hypothesis of TMS effects rather than showing separate storage of the timing of execution and other parameters. Consistent with Day et al., increasing TMS intensity increases the delay in the saccade (see figure 5.7), and applying TMS close in time to the expected onset of the saccade (−50 to −80 msec) produced longer delays than using earlier pulse times (−80 to −110 msec). Express saccades, which are not cortically driven, were unaffected by the TMS, but auditorily cued saccades were disrupted in the same way as visually guided

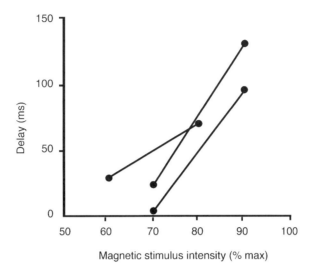

Figure 5.7   Increasing the intensity of TMS increases the delays induced in saccadic-onset latency. Data are from three individual subjects, intensity is expressed as a percentage of stimulator output (MagStim 200). (From Priori et al., 1993, with permission.)

eye movements. Similar results were obtained by Zangmeister, Canavan, and
Hoemberg (1995), who used more focal TMS over the parietal cortex and reported an effect on accuracy and acceleration of saccades when TMS was
applied to the PPC or the prefrontal cortex. Critically, they found that stimulation approximately 70 msec before saccade onset had greater effects than stimulation 20 msec before onset. Thus, between the two studies, the critical time to
apply TMS to disrupt eye movements has been bracketed at approximately
60–80 msec prior to saccade onset, a factor that needs to be taken into account
in physiological and computational models.

Memory-guided saccades also seem to depend on the PPC, and TMS applied over the right but not the left PPC can interfere with a saccade to a remembered location in either right or left visual space (Oyachi and Ohtsuka, 1995).
In contrast to Priori et al. (1993), Oyachi and Ohtsuka's study observed a large
cost in accuracy, but less so in latency, and they suggested that the "TMS pulse

may activate LIP cells for short periods and change the motor planning but it does not abolish the signal." This dissociation between saccade memory and execution does not mean that the two are stored separately in space; it rather suggests that they occupy different segments of time in the processes carried out by the parietal cortex.

The role of the parietal cortex in memory-guided saccades has been investigated further by Muri and colleagues (1996, 2000), who found the left PPC to be important but at a later time than the right PPC and, unlike Oyachi and Ohtsuka, obtained a delay in saccadic latency as a result of TMS. Terao et al. (1998b) used TMS to assess the relative timing of two cortical regions, one between 2–4 cm anterior and 2–4 cm lateral of the motor hand area (a site they suggest overlies the frontal eye fields) and a second 6–8 cm posterior and 0–4 cm lateral to the hand area (a site they called the PPC). In the critical conditions, subjects were given single-pulse TMS at 80, 100, or 120 msec after onset of a cue to make a saccade away from a target. They used an antisaccade task because there were no effects of TMS on visually guided saccades in their pilot experiments. However, TMS did delay saccade onset in the antisaccade paradigm when applied at 80 msec over the PPC and at 100 msec when applied over the frontal eye fields. There was no apparent difference in the character of deficits caused by frontal eye field or PPC stimulation, but an interesting pattern emerged when the results obtained with different dependent variables were compared. When latencies were taken as the outcome measure, stimulation to either hemisphere caused latency increases irrespective of the direction of the saccade. When prosaccades (errors in the form of saccades toward the target rather than away) were counted, however, stimulation of the right hemisphere caused prosaccades to the left, and TMS of the left hemisphere caused saccades to the right. The prosaccades were induced by TMS of the occipital cortex, the anterior or posterior parietal cortex, and the motor cortex as well as the FEFs, and they were induced mainly by early (80 msec) rather than later (100 or 120 msec) applications of TMS. Terao et al.'s results suggest a simple feedforward model of cortical activity in antisaccades, but it is not clear whether the prosaccades were caused by errors in the eye movement system or by a nonspecific effect that prevented inhibition of the visual target. Resolving the differences between these experiments in the domain of eye movements will rest on further studies of the parietal cortex and on establishing the role of frontal areas in visual and memory-guided eye movements (Zangmeister, Canavan, and Hoemberg, 1995; Muri et al., 2000).

SEQUENCING TIME: GETTING THINGS IN ORDER

In addition to studies of visual perception, single-pulse TMS has been used in studies of motor behavior to delineate a chain of events from movement selection in the premotor cortex, execution by the motor cortex, and error correction by the PPC. Patients with lesions of the left premotor areas may be apraxic and have difficulty selecting movements, and it has been argued that the left hemisphere is responsible for the selection of actions (Kimura and Archibald, 1974; Kimura, 1993; Rushworth, Ellison, and Walsh, 2001). It is difficult to demonstrate that the reason why a patient is poor at making accurate movements is that they are poor at selecting the appropriate movement rather than that they lack coordination, for example, and it remains a major challenge to probe the timing of interactions between areas.

Rushworth and colleagues used single-pulse TMS to segregate the timing and location of selection from the timing and location of execution (Schluter et al., 1998, 1999). Subjects were presented with a conditional visual cue and were required to respond by pressing a key with an index finger if presented with a large square or a small rectangle and with the middle finger of the same hand if presented with a small circle or a large rectangle. TMS was applied at cue—TMS asynchronies of 0–340 msec over the anterior premotor cortex, the posterior premotor cortex, and the motor cortex contralateral to the responding hand. As figure 5.8 shows, TMS over the anterior premotor cortex delayed response time if it was applied approximately 140 msec after visual cue onset, whereas TMS over the motor cortex delayed activity only if applied between 220 and 300 msec after visual cue onset. TMS at the intermediate site was effective in increasing response time if applied at an intermediate time (180 msec).

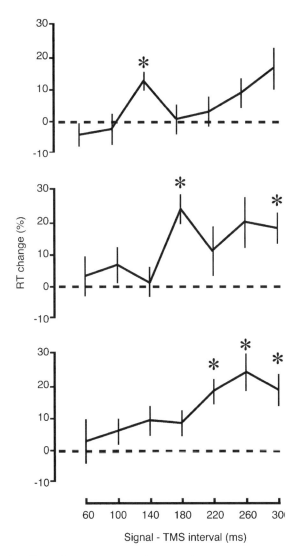

Figure 5.8   The effects of TMS on motor selection. Subjects were required to make one of two motor responses contingent on the combination of size and form in a visual cue. TMS applied over the premotor cortex to disrupt response selection increased reaction times if applied approximately 140 msec after the cue (*top diagram*). TMS over the motor cortex, which disrupted execution rather than selection, had maximal effect when applied closer to the time of response, 220 msec or more after the visual cue (*bottom diagram*). TMS over a site intermediate between the premotor and the motor cortex (*middle diagram*) delayed reaction times when applied at a time later than effective TMS of the premotor cortex and earlier than TMS of motor cortex, perhaps by disrupting information transfer between the sites of selection and execution.

The interpretation of these data is that the earlier TMS effects reflect a disruption of early processes such as selection and later TMS effects reflect disruption of execution. The case was strengthened by the novel demonstration that TMS over the left premotor cortex also disrupted selection of actions for the *ipsilateral* hand, but ipsilateral effects were not seen for right premotor stimulation or for any motor cortex stimulation. Thus, the left premotor cortex is required for selecting actions for both left and right motor areas.

The sequence of virtual-lesion effects from selection to action in an anterior to posterior direction was extended by Desmurget et al. (1999). One can select actions and execute them but as anyone who has wielded a tennis racquet or baseball bat knows, some shots have to be corrected on line as the ball bounces or swerves unexpectedly. Desmurget et al. presented subjects with LEDs at varying eccentricities from fixation and applied TMS as the subjects reached out to touch the lights. On critical trials, the location of the light was changed by 7.5 degrees after the subjects had begun their arm movement, and TMS was applied over the left PPC at the time this movement began. On non-TMS trials, subjects corrected perfectly well for changes in the position of the LED even though they were unaware of the change in its position. TMS had little or no effect on the speed of the subjects' movements but had significant effects, making the subjects' errors larger, on positional correction for the shifted LED. The effect was specific to the arm contralateral to the hemisphere receiving TMS.

The premotor cortex does not select all actions, however. It appears that eye movements are selected at a site anterior to the premotor cortex, the frontal eye fields, as shown in monkeys with frontal eye field lesions (Collin et al., 1982), and it remains to be seen, using single-pulse TMS, whether the two systems—selecting for eye movements and selecting for body movements—have similar time courses or patterns of interference when there is a conflict of information.

Differences between motor areas also have been highlighted with respect to motor task difficulty. Gerloff et al. (1997) compared the effects of 15–20 Hz rTMS over primary motor, posterior parietal, and supplementary motor cortices while subjects played overlearned sequences of different complexity on a keyboard. Stimulation over the primary motor cortex contralateral to the hand pressing the keys, as one would expect, significantly disturbed performance when subjects were playing either a simple scale or a complex sequence. Only the more complex sequence, however, was disrupted by supplementary motor stimulation. No errors were induced by TMS over frontal (EEG sites FCz, F3, F4) or parietal (sites CPz, P3, P4) cortices. Gerloff et al. argue that this is evidence for a role of the SMA in organizing future events in complex sequences. However, the errors following SMA stimulation occur later than those caused by TMS of the motor cortex, whereas a planning hypothesis would predict that the SMA effects should occur earlier, so one can conclude from this study only that the SMA is more important in complex rather than simple sequences. To test the conclusion that the SMA has an organizing role, a single-pulse investigation is required to show that TMS over the SMA impairs complex rather than simple sequences and that the critical time of effective TMS occurs earlier in the SMA than in the motor cortex, similar to the results reported by Schluter et al. (1998, 1999). Such controls are important. Otherwise, the finding that TMS to a given cortical region disrupts performance in complex rather than simple tasks cannot rule out nonspecific distracting effects of TMS and can provide false-positive results.

Actions, even once selected, are not simple unitary phenomena to investigate. The simple act of reaching to pick up a cup requires reach, grasp, and lift components and different phases within each. It would be both elegant and ecologically valid if the action could undergo empirical parsing in a single experiment. Lemon, Johansson, and Westling (1995) carried out an experiment in which a task was broken up into different analyzable stages without being interrupted. EMG recordings were elicited from several different muscles as subjects reached out to lift a small object. This simple task was broken down into eight segments (midreach, late reach, pretouch, touch, load, transitional, lift, and hold), and EMGs were recorded at all these different phases. The pattern of changes in the EMG depended on the recording site and on the phase of the action but was not a simple reflection of the muscular activity required at any given phase. Figure 5.9 shows the recordings from just two of the muscle sites (first dorsal interosseous and brachioradialis). The application of TMS here is not as a lesion,

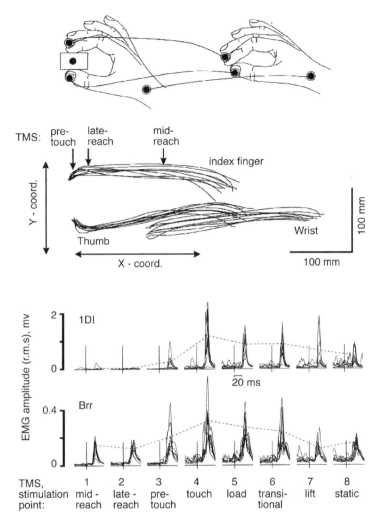

Figure 5.9 Kinematics of the reach during the reach–lift task used by Lemon, Johansson, and Westling (1995). Data were from markers placed on the top of the object to be lifted, the nail of the index finger, nail of the thumb, and the wrist (*first panel,* at top of figure). At the onset of each trial, the hand rested on the subject's knee, and TMS was applied during different phases of the action of raising the hand to reach out and lift the object: during midreach, late–reach, or pretouch phases (*second panel*). The traces in the second panel show the trajectories of the reaches without TMS. The third and fourth panels show EMG traces from the first dorsal interosseous (1DI) and the brachioradialis (Brr) evoked by TMS during different phases of the task. Nine trials, one subject. Vertical lines on each trace mark the timing of TMS.

but as an on-line recorder of corticospinal modulation of muscle activity during a task performed naturally.

Sensitivity to touch has received less attention than motor behavior in TMS studies, but the few studies available on the subject show that the somatosensory cortex is a rich, relatively untapped vein for the technique. As with motor cortex stimulation, one can produce an output of the somatosensory cortex in the form of paresthesias (Amassian et al., 1991; Cohen et al., 1991), but more interesting possibilities lie in the virtual-lesion approach. Cohen et al. (1991d) induced a decrease in sensitivity of the fingers contralateral to the side of stimulation; this finding forms the basis of two studies that have looked at the relationship of the two hemispheres in cutaneous perception. Seyal, Ro, and Rafal (1995) tested the proposal that extinction is a function of abnormal interactions between the two cerebral hemispheres (Cohen et al., 1994). Damage to one of the parietal lobes can result in disinhibition of the intact hemisphere, which leads to the prediction that patients should show not only a decreased efficiency in orienting attention in space contralateral to the lesion but also an increased efficiency in orienting in ipsilesional space. Seyal, Ro, and Rafal's subjects carried out a tactile-detection task with the thumb of the hand ipsilateral to the site of stimulation and received single-pulse TMS 50 msec prior to the delivery of the electrical stimulus they had to detect with the thumb. In trials without TMS or with TMS over the frontal cortex, subjects detected a mean of 18% of thumb stimulations, but detected 50% when TMS was delivered over the parietal cortex (3–5 cm posterior to the somatosensory cortex). Methodologically this result is intriguing because it presents a rare case of TMS being applied before the sensory stimulus; if we are to understand the effective duration of TMS interference, we should in principle be able to bracket the deficits produced by single-pulse TMS with stimulation both before and after presentation of the discriminanda (see figure 3.16). Improving performance on a task that subjects found so difficult to perform (18% correct) is difficult to interpret, however, and the detection performance of the subjects was "elevated" only to chance levels by TMS. Seyal, Ro, and Rafal, therefore produced psychometric functions of detections at different intensities of the cutaneous stimulation. Relative to TMS over the frontal cortex or the motor cortex, there was a leftward shift in the function following right parietal TMS, but it is not clear whether the effect would be robust on tasks in which subjects can peform at a higher level.

Oliveri et al. (1999a, 1999b) also have examined interactions between the hemispheres. TMS was applied 4 cm anterior (frontal site) or 4 cm posterior (parietal site) to the motor hand area, and subjects were required to detect electrical stimulation of one of three digits on either hand. Unlike Seyal, Ro, and Rafal's experiment, the magnetic stimulation was delivered at 20 or 40 msec after presentation of the sensory stimulation and could be applied to either hand individually or both hands simultaneously. Right-hemisphere TMS led to a small increase in errors (less than 5%) irrespective of whether the TMS was applied to the parietal or frontal site, whether the finger stimulation was unimanual or bimanual, and whether the right or left hand was stimulated; that is, right-hemisphere TMS disrupted tactile perception with right and left hands, rather than having an enhancing effect in the ipsilateral hand. The authors concluded that the right parietal cortex has a predominant role in bilateral cutaneous perception.

There are several possible sources for Oliveri et al.'s and Seyal et al.'s conflicting conclusions. In their experiment, Oliveri et al. stimulated at 100% of motor threshold, 20 or 40 msec after sensory stimulation, tested both hands and both hemispheres under unimanual and bimanual conditions, and measured errors in a relatively easy task. Seyal et al. used 110% of threshold, 50 msec before sensory stimulation, and tested only one hand and one hemisphere under ipsilateral stimulation. We already have suggested that criterion changes cannot be excluded as an explanation of Seyal et al.'s results, but the procedural differences between their experiment and Oliveri et al.'s experiment suggest other possibilities. The lower TMS intensity used by Oliveri et al. may have been insufficient to cause interhemispheric disinhibition—a proposal that is easily tested. Another testable option is that the later magnetic stimulation times used by Oliveri et al. were too late to allow expression of a disinhibition effect. Recall that Ilmoniemi et al.'s (1997) EEG data (chapter 3) showed that the initial effects of TMS are strongest at the site of stimulation and that effects on anatomically connected sites can take several tens of milliseconds to emerge.

So far we have dealt with studies of the motor system or visual system in isolation, but the goal of the brain is behavior, and a researcher might reasonably think of one of the major outputs of the visual system as something that is of use to the motor system (Milner and Goodale, 1995). There are several notable examples of how TMS can be used to scrutinize the interactions of visual-to-motor information processing. Marzi et al. (1998), for example, revealed the timing of visuomotor information transfer between the two cerebral hemispheres. Subjects were presented with a single visual cue in one of the two visual hemifields and made a single key press response with a designated hand. TMS was applied at one time point (targeted at extrastriate visual cortex due to lack of callosal connections between the striate cortex in each hemisphere) 50 msec after the onset of the visual cue and was seen to delay the key press if the cue was presented in the hemifield ipsilateral to the responding hand—that is, if the information had to cross the callosum. Zangaladze et al. (1999) exposed an even closer link between visual and tactile systems—that one is necessary to the other. Their study was motivated by previous TMS work on plasticity (Pascual-Leone and Torres, 1993; Cohen et al., 1997), to which we return in chapter 7. Subjects were given tactile detection and discrimination tasks and received TMS over the *visual* cortex. Remarkably, TMS interfered with the ability to discriminate tactile orientations if it was applied 180 msec after stimulus presentation. The temporal sampling in this experiment was sparse, and it would be interesting to see TMS delivered at many more times, particularly to facilitate a comparison between the effects of TMS and the timing of responses to tactile orientation in visual area V4 (Haenny, Maunsell, and Schiller, 1988).

TIME ON ONE'S HANDS

Visual imagery is a function one might consider to be dominated by visual cortex (see discussion of Kosslyn et al., 1993a, 1993b, 1999 in chapter 6). However, which brain areas are involved depends on what is being rotated, and imaging studies have generated a debate regarding the role of primary motor cortex in mental rotation of pictures of hands (see Kosslyn 1998). Ganis et al. (2000)

applied single-pulse TMS to the hand representation of the motor cortex while subjects made same/different judgments on the orientation of images of hands or feet. Pulses were applied at either 400 or 650 msec (the times selected on the basis of MEG data [Kawamichi et al., 1998]), and they increased reaction times to mentally rotate the hands but not the feet when delivered at 400 msec but not at 650 msec (figure 5.10). This stimulus specificity of the role of the motor cortex is intriguing because the visual processes involved in mental rotation would be completed before the involvement of motor cortex.

Earlier work also demonstrated a link between imagery and motor activity. Fadiga et al. (1999) measured MEPs from the hand muscles contralateral to the hemisphere of stimulation while subjects were either imagining or actually opening or closing their hand. The MEPs recorded during imagery mimicked those recorded during real movements. Fadiga et al. then applied TMS to the motor cortex during imagery, and the resulting MEPs revealed a facilitatory effect restricted to the hemisphere contralateral to the imagined hand (see also Fadiga et al., 1995). Observing movements also can change the excitability of the cortex. Strafella and Paus (2000) applied paired-pulse TMS over the motor cortex during rest, while subjects observed hand writing and while they observed arm movements. Observing actions increased the amplitude of the MEP and decreased paired-pulse inhibition, and these changes were specific to the muscle involved. For example, with a 3 msec interstimulus interval, MEPs recorded from the first dorsal interosseous increased when subjects viewed a hand movement but not an arm movement, and MEPs recorded from the biceps increased when subjects viewed an arm but not a hand movement.

TIME PRESENT: CATCHING THE BRAIN (UN)AWARE

Awareness of events is, like any other psychological phenomena, subject to the temporal sequences of brain processes and therefore invites investigation with single-pulse TMS. There are at least three questions here: When are we aware of events? Which brain regions are responsible? And what are the interactions between these areas? The questions are closely linked, of course, but by dividing

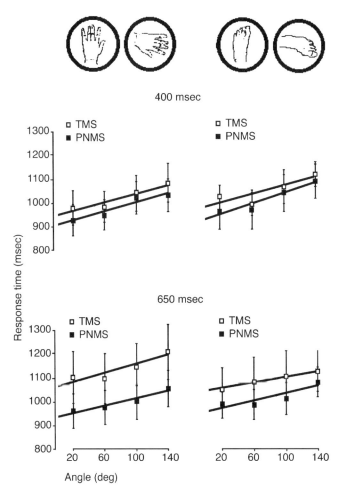

Figure 5.10   TMS and hand rotation. Average reaction times plotted as a function of angle of rotation difference between stimuli (hands or feet) to be matched as same or different. Open squares, reaction times for motor cortex stimulation; filled squares, reaction times for peripheral nerve magnetic stimulation (PNMS). Upper two histograms show data for a visual stimulus—TMS asynchrony of 400 msec; lower histograms show data for a stimulus—TMS asynchrony of 650 msec. (From Ganis et al., 2000, with permission.)

them in this way the scientific approach to awareness has in a few short years proved more fruitful than the philosophers' longstanding approach of wondering what awareness might really *be*.

An apparently simple observation is that people tend to think they have moved before measurements of muscle responses indicate they have done so, and this experience of having moved is almost 100 msec ahead of the movement (Libet et al., 1983). Quite apart from the reassurance one might get from knowing one's brain is such a long way ahead of one's actions, Libet et al.'s observation generates hypotheses about the where and what of awareness. Haggard and Magno (1999) contrasted the roles of the premotor cortex and the primary motor cortex in awareness of action by giving a single pulse of TMS over one of these areas after subjects had been cued to respond to a tone. Here the response reaction time wasn't the only dependent variable of interest; subjects also were asked to indicate on a clock face precisely *when* they thought they had responded. TMS applied over the frontal site (electrode location FCz) produced a greater delay in subjects' perception of when they had responded relative to when they actually had responded. The opposite pattern was the case with TMS over M1; subjects' experienced time of response was much less delayed relative to the delay in actual reaction time (figure 5.11). This asymmetry of effects led Haggard and Magno to conclude that awareness of action is generated, at least in part, somewhere between the premotor and the primary motor cortex. Just as important as this partial localization of awareness is the hint of the *contents* of awareness. This experiment suggests that it is not actions one is aware of, but the intention to make them. Haggard and Magno put it more conservatively: "our awareness of movement is at least partly an awareness of premotor process" (1999, 107). But if we have an idea about what premotor cortex may be crucial for, as discussed earlier (Schluter et al., 1998, 1999), we also can go as far as to say what awareness of its processes might be. A crucial matter here is the lateralization of awareness. Rushworth and colleagues (1998) showed that left premotor cortex was important for selection of actions for both left and right motor cortex, and Haggard and Magno have shown the importance of stimulating around premotor areas. The round coil over FCz (the direction of current is unspecified) means that premotor areas in both hemipheres may have received

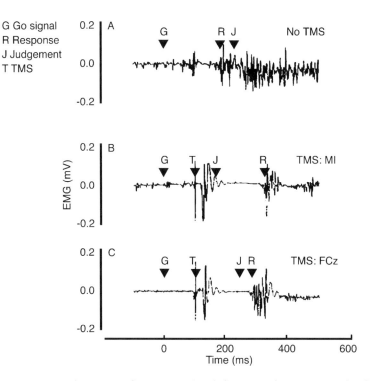

Figure 5.11   TMS and awareness of action. Typical trials from one subject in a control trial in which the subject responds to an auditory imperative cue and judges the time, from a visual cue, at which the subject believed himself to have pressed the response button. (*A*) Control trial without TMS: the subject judges the time of response (judged time 230 msec) to be slightly later than the onset of EMG increases recorded from the first dorsal interosseous (184 msec). (*B*) TMS applied over the motor cortex 100 msec after the imperative signal produced a large MEP. The subject's response was delayed substantially (327 msec), but the subject's judgment of when the response was made was close to the time without TMS (169 msec). (*C*) TMS over a frontal midline site also evoked an MEP and delayed response time (283 msec), and the judged time also was delayed (243 msec). (From Haggard and Magno, 1999, with permission.)

magnetic stimulation. This lack of specificity leaves untested the prediction one can make from Rushworth et al.'s experiments that, to the extent awareness of action is awareness of premotor processes, TMS over the left premotor cortex should have a greater effect than TMS over the right premotor cortex.

Awareness of what one does is one matter; awareness of what one sees is another. A long-running debate regarding visual awareness centers around whether area V1 is necessary or whether functionally specialized areas such as V4 and V5 are sufficient for awareness of the visual attribute for which they are relatively specialized. As we saw in chapter 4, stimulation over extrastriate cortical area V5 of sighted subjects yields a perception of movement (Stewart et al., 1999; Hotson et al., 1994), and stimulation of V1—or, more correctly, the occipital pole—produces the sensation of stationary phosphenes. In addressing the problem of visual awareness, Cowey and Walsh (2000) induced phosphenes by TMS to examine the integrity of the visual cortex in a totally retinally blind subject and to compare the results with those obtained by stimulating the same regions in normally sighted individuals and in an hemianopic subject who possesses blindsight in the impaired field. Vivid phosphenes were elicited easily from the blind subject when TMS was applied to the occipital pole and moving phosphenes when TMS was applied to V5 (figure 5.12). However, extensive and intensive stimulation of the damaged hemisphere in the blindsight subject did not yield reliable or reproducible phosphenes—even when applied to an intact area V5 on that side. Thus, the experience of the motion seems to depend upon the integrity of striate cortex (Cowey and Walsh, 2000; Pascual-Leone and Walsh, 2001).

Pascual-Leone and Walsh (2001) probed the timing of the interactions between V5 and V1 by stimulating the occipital pole a few milliseconds after stimulating V5. First of all, phosphenes were elicited in overlapping regions of the visual field by stimulation of V5 or the striate cortex, and the phosphene threshold for these regions was established. Single-pulse TMS was then applied to V5 at 100% of phosphene threshold and over the occipital pole at 80% of phosphene threshold. When the two pulses were delivered together, subjects reliably reported the perception of a moving phosphene, but as the asynchrony of V5 and V1 TMS increased, the confidence of the subjects diminished, and they reported either stationary phosphenes or were unsure of the direction of

V1 Phosphenes

Single pulse;
70% of output
Midline & lateral
above inion

(a)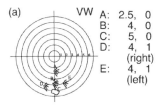

VW

A:	2.5,	0
B:	4,	0
C:	5,	0
D:	4,	1
	(right)	
E:	4,	1
	(left)	

5Hz, 0.5 sec
80% of output
Midline and lateral
above inion

(b)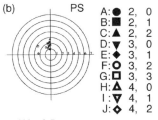

PS

A:●	2,	0
B:■	2,	1
C:▲	2,	2
D:▼	3,	0
E:◆	3,	1
F:○	3,	2
G:□	3,	3
H:△	4,	0
I:▽	4,	1
J:◇	4,	2

8Hz, 0.5 sec
70% of output
Right hemisphere
Midline and lateral
above inion

(c)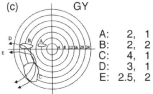

GY

A:	2,	1
B:	2,	2
C:	4,	1
D:	3,	1
E:	2.5,	2

V5 Phosphenes

10 Hz, 0.5 sec;
70% of output
Midline & lateral
above inion

(a)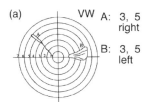

VW

A: 3, 5
right

B: 3, 5
left

5Hz, 0.5 sec
80% of output
Midline and lateral
above inion

(b)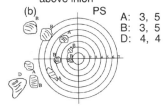

PS

A: 3, 5
B: 3, 5
D: 4, 4

80% of output
Right hemisphere
Midline and lateral
above inion

(c)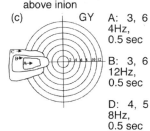

GY

A: 3, 6
4Hz,
0.5 sec

B: 3, 6
12Hz,
0.5 sec

D: 4, 5
8Hz,
0.5 sec

movement when TMS was applied over V1 between 5 and 15 msec after TMS over V5. When TMS was applied over the occipital pole 15–45 msec after the pulse delivered to V5, the perception of the phosphene was abolished. To discount the possibility of the effects being due to disrupting fast feed-forward projections to V5 from V1, Pascual-Leone and Walsh used the same procedure with double stimulation of V5, and, consistent with the backprojection hypothesis there was no effect of the second TMS pulse on the phosphene produced by the first pulse (figure 5.13). This finding reflects the time window of the back projection from V5 to V1 and is consistent with recent studies of cortical deactivation in monkeys in which cooling of extrastriate areas decreases the sensitivity of neurons in V1 (see Bullier 2001 for review). This experiment is also a good example of the effects even apparently low levels of TMS can have on cortical functioning: The neural noise induced need not be great if the task, the timing of TMS, and the sites of stimulation are optimized.

TIME FUTURE: TEMPORAL ASYNCHRONY IN PERCEPTION

The temporal properties of TMS have only begun to be used in earnest. The relative timing of events have yet to be explored in language functions,

Figure 5.12 Phosphenes elicited by occipital TMS (*a*) in a normally sighted observer (*b*) in peripherally blind subject P.S., and (*c*) in hemianopic patient G.Y. The coordinates give the site of stimulation in dorsal-lateral order. For example, 2,1 indicates that the coil was centered 2 cm above the inion and 1 cm lateral. Note that as the coil is moved superiorly away from the inion, the phosphenes migrate inferiorly (e.g., phosphenes A and C in G.Y.'s bottom left plot [*left c*]), and that as the coil is moved away from the midline the phosphenes migrate farther into the contralateral visual field (e.g., phospenes A and B in G.Y.'s bottom right plot 1 [*right c*]). In subject P.S., the phosphenes remain resolutely in the central few degrees of the visual field despite stimulation being delivered between 2 and 5 cm above the inion and up to 2 cm lateral. Where there are phosphenes elicited beyond the central two degrees for this subject, they are in the opposite direction to that predicted by normal retinotopic mapping (stimulating more superiorly will yield more superior phosphenes than inferior phosphenes). Moving phosphenes are shown in the three right-hand figures, (*a*) in a normally sighted observer, (*b*) in peripherally blind subject P.S., and (*c*) in hemianopic patient G.Y. All three subjects reported moving phosphenes.

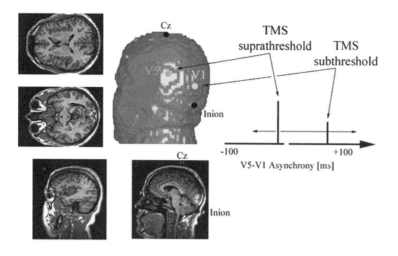

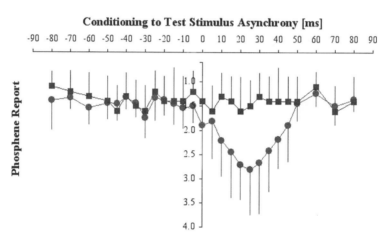

Figure 5.13 (*Top*) Schematic representation of the experimental design of a V5-V1 interaction study. The brain MRI image from one of the study subjects displays a representative example of the site of stimulation for induction of stationary (V1) and moving phosphenes (MT+/V5). The location on the subject's scalp of the center of the intersection of the wings in the figure-of-eight TMS coil is projected, perpendicularly to the scalp surface, onto the subject's brain as reconstructed from an anatomical MRI. (*Bottom*) Mean responses of all subjects ($n = 8$) to combined stimulation of V5 and V1. The V5-V1-TMS asynchrony is displayed on the *x*-axis: negative values indicate that V1 received TMS prior to V5, and positive values indicate that V1 was stimulated after V5. The subjects made one of four judgments. (1) The phosphene elicited by V5 TMS was present and moving; (2) the phosphene was present, but the subject was not confident to judge whether moving; (3) the phosphene was present but stationary; (4) no phosphene was observed. TMS over V1 between 10 and 30 msec after TMS over V5 affected the perception of the phosphene (see text for details).

memory, priming, and many other domains, including the perception of time itself. There is no doubt that an explanation of how it is we perceive a unified world will require an understanding of how the brain constructs temporal order, and there are already candidates presented clearly enough for experimentation. Moutoussis and Zeki (1997) have argued that awareness of change in the color domain is up to 80 msec faster than awareness of change of visual motion direction. This is a counterintuitive claim given that the motion system is temporally transient and faster than the sustained, slower color system. The finding has been replicated in principle; however, in this case color awareness was found to be only 7 msec ahead of awareness of motion (Barbur et al., 1999). A development of Haggard and Magno's (1999) paradigm may be a way to begin to interfere with the apparently segregated awareness of different visual attributes. If one were to use Moutoussis and Zeki's paradigm, for example, the timing of evoked potentials and EMG responses may be compared with the subjects' estimation of when they saw the color or direction of movement change. The difference between estimated awareness and evoked activity may provide a time window through which TMS can effect a disruption of awareness without any effects on accuracy. Other candidate explanations abound. Amassian et al. have argued that the frontal lobe is the origin of visual awareness by "opening a thalamic gate for brief parietal or occipital outputs, which then reach consciousness" (1998). Many of the areas proposed to be important for visual awareness by different authors—V1, extrastriate visual cortex, parietal cortex, and frontal lobe—are accessible to TMS in humans; even more are on the lateral surface of the cortex in nonhuman primates. Clearly, TMS still has much to contribute to chronometric analyses of perceptual integration and awareness.

CHRONOMETRIC IMPOSSIBILITIES?

The assumption underlying our discussion of virtual-lesion effect up to this point has been that the time window of neural processes can always be identified. This assumption might be wrong not only in practice but also in principle, and there may be some processes or some areas that carry out multiple functions in a task or, in other words, that cannot be parsed into discrete units (Miller, 1988). Where information transmission is continuous rather than discrete, for example, it is difficult to see how single-pulse TMS can be used to yield a neurochronometric picture. The distinction between self-contained information-processing units and spatially or temporally overlapping processes is, like many dichotomies, likely to be blurred toward a continuum and to vary according to the elements required to perform the task, the similarities between alternative outcomes, the experience of the subject, and the difficulty of the task. Continuous involvement of an area in a task has been suggested at several different levels of the information-processing hierarchies. Schall and colleagues, for example, have proposed that the frontal cortex is involved continuously in visual search (Bichot et al., in press), and Walsh et al. (1998b) have made a similar suggestion for area V5 (MT) in tasks that require selective filtering of movement. This involvement has two consequences for TMS studies, both of which provide empirical challenges that can be met by TMS but not by other methods. Where an area is involved continuously in a task, one may resort to applying rTMS across the whole period of the task. This would assume, however, that because an area is involved—let's say, for 2,000 msec—its function is iterative across that period. The assumption is unwarranted: Continuity does not imply uniformity; it is just as likely that what an area contributes to a task in the first 500 msec is different from the demands it must meet in the last 500 msec. If this were so, then one might predict different consequences of TMS applied in the early and late phases of a task. For example, TMS in the first 500 msec may induce errors in a task, whereas TMS in the last 500 msec may induce reaction-time costs. A second consequence is that continuous involvement of one area may be predictive of continuous involvement of other areas with which it is connected, which immediately allows one to make predictions based on the interactions of different cortical areas. Continuous involvement, then, is not a bar to neurochronometry; it is a source of hypotheses. The time windows of neurochronometry do not lie solely in the gift of single-pulse TMS, and in chapter 6 we show how rTMS has been used to parse neurocognitive processes with relatively broader temporal windows.

DYNAMIC NEUROPSYCHOLOGY: REPETITIVE-PULSE TMS

TIME IS NOT ALWAYS OF THE ESSENCE

In discussing the potential of single-pulse TMS, we highlighted the temporal resolution of the technique and contrasted this resolution with the lack of temporal information in studies of neuropsychological patients. It is the most salient advantage of TMS, but it may give the unintended impression that single-pulse TMS *must* be used for fine chronometry or that rTMS cannot add to neuropsychology other than by replicating deficits. Single-pulse TMS has uses that do not depend on teasing apart functions that occur a few milliseconds apart, and the functional resolution of rTMS is such that it opens a new window onto brain function—one that stands between the windows opened by single-pulse TMS and neuropsychological studies. It is an error to imagine that rTMS does not have good temporal resolution, an error that can lead one to underestimate its potential. The stimulation duration used in rTMS studies is usually between 500 and 1,000 msec, which is still a very short period for reversible intervention and still too short for new cognitive strategies to be employed or for any brain reorganization to occur. The problem space revealed by this type of intermediate temporal precision is well suited to studying dynamic interactions between areas involved in specific cognitive functions. In this chapter, we look at ways in which single-pulse TMS and rTMS have been used in cognitive studies that do not depend on fine temporal resolution: modeling the effects of lesions, testing hypotheses generated by imaging studies, and producing paradoxical functional facilitations. In all three areas, TMS has advanced knowledge within meaningful theoretical frameworks.

MAKING MODELS: IT'S WORTH PAYING ATTENTION

Replicating effects seen in patients is a good starting point for a TMS study. It also may be a good end. Replication is rarely exact, and the differences between real and virtual patients can be important and informative. In the first demonstration of attentional effects with rTMS, Pascual-Leone and colleagues (1994b) applied 25 Hz TMS over the occipital, parietal, or temporal cortices. The aim was to study a well-known phenomenon, visual extinction, which most often is seen following right parietal lesions. Subjects showing extinction can detect and identify targets that are presented singly in one or other of the two visual fields but are unable to detect the stimulus in the field contralateral to the lesion if the two stimuli are presented together. In Pascual-Leone et al.'s study, stimulation of the right parietal cortex duly reproduced visual extinction of left visual field stimuli when two targets were presented. But stimulation of the left parietal cortex also produced the phenomenon with equal facility (figure 6.1). As expected, occipital stimulation interfered with the perception of any stimuli contralateral to the hemisphere that received TMS, and no clear effects were seen with temporal cortex stimulation. The difference between the real and virtual patients can be accounted for by considering reorganization following brain damage. From this experiment, one might conclude that both hemispheres are balanced equally in the competition for attention to visual areas, and the predominance of the right hemisphere, inferred from extinction studies of neuropsychological patients, is due to an advantage in reorganization of the left hemisphere.

Modeling of visual neglect by Fierro et al. (2000) reinforces the common view that the right hemisphere does have a special role in visuospatial orienting. Neglect is widely studied in neuropsychological patients, but there are many

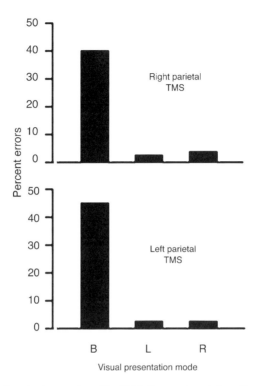

Figure 6.1   Visual extinction produced by TMS. Data replotted from Pascual-Leone et al., 1994. When two stimuli are presented simultaneously (one in each hemifield, indicated as B on the abscissae), TMS over the parietal lobe reduces detection of the stimulus in the contralateral visual field to chance levels. Detection is not reduced when single stimuli are presented to one hemifield (L or R).

differences between patients, and the tendency is for the phenomenon to be transient (Bisiach and Vallar, 1988). By taking a psychophysical approach, Fierro et al. have produced a protocol that may be useful in modeling neglect. Subjects were presented briefly (50 msec) with prebisected lines and required to judge whether the left, right, or neither side was longer. In control trials, there was a pseudoneglect tendency, consistent with right-hemisphere bias, to report the left as longer (Bowers and Heilman, 1980; McCourt and Jewell, 1999). On TMS

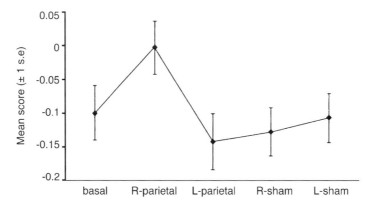

Figure 6.2   The effect of TMS on the perception of bisected lines. When TMS is applied to the right parietal cortex, subjects judged the relative lengths of the two sides of bisected lines relatively well (zero represents perfect discrimination). Without TMS, the subjects showed a right pseudoneglect and judged the left sides of the lines to be longer than they were. TMS over left parietal cortex had no effect on this pseudoneglect, nor did sham TMS over left or right parietal cortex. In principle, this correction of a pseudoneglect may provide a basis for modeling the neglect suffered by neuropsychological patients. (From Fierro et al., 2000, with permission.)

trials, pulses were delivered at 115% of motor threshold at 25 Hz for 400 msec over the left or right parietal cortex at the time of stimulus onset. Right parietal stimulation corrected the pseudoneglect, but left parietal and sham TMS did not change the subjects' behavior (figure 6.2). The ability to reproduce neglect is an important step in modeling the phenomenon, and one wonders whether a re-action time or signal detection approach might increase the sensitivity of this particular assay.

NECESSITY AND SUFFICIENCY: BLINDING THE MIND'S EYE

There are many instances of lesion studies being in apparent conflict with single-unit physiology or brain-imaging results. These disagreements often are caused by different experimental conditions being used with the two tech-niques or by a lack of overlap between the spatiotemporal properties of the two techniques and thus a debate being carried out across a divide between two different problem spaces (cf. figure 1.1). The solution often has to come from another technical avenue. The role of primary visual area V1 in visual imagery has been one such dispute. When subjects are asked to use depictive imagery, blood flow in area V1 is increased relative to a condition in which no visual stimuli are presented and visual imagination is not required. The question is whether imagery depends on V1 (Kosslyn, 1988; Kosslyn et al., 1993a, 1993b) or if the activity seen is epiphenomenal or not representative of visuotopic processing in imagery.

To investigate this question, Kosslyn et al. (1999) used identical task conditions in a rTMS study and in a PET experiment. In the TMS experiment, subjects received 1 Hz stimulation at 90% of motor threshold for 5 min. They then were required to visualize and compare the properties of memorized images of grating patterns or of real images of the same stimuli. The reaction times of subjects were increased significantly in both real perception and imagery conditions (see figure 6.3), showing that area V1 was critical for visual imagery as well as for perception. The effect of TMS was greater for imagery than for real perception, which may reflect the fact that the imagery condition was more difficult than the perception condition.

In Kosslyn et al.'s experiment, TMS was not applied *during* the task but *before* it (see the discussion of distal TMS in chapter 4). Previous work had shown that slow trains of rTMS could decrease cortical excitability for several minutes after the stimulation had ceased (Chen et al., 1997a; Pascual-Leone et al., 1998b). It is clear that at the present time one cannot say that stimulation parameters that have a behavioral effect in one domain will necessarily work in another. If a set of stimulation parameters produces effects on a particular task, all one can say is that those parameters work for that task and that brain area in conjunction. For example, 1 Hz for 5 min over the striate cortex may be sufficient to prevent any compensatory adaptation to TMS effects that would assist visual imagery, but such recovery as might occur might be sufficient for normal performance of another task—it depends on the redundancy of capacity for the given task. As such, the consequences of distal TMS over the occipital visual

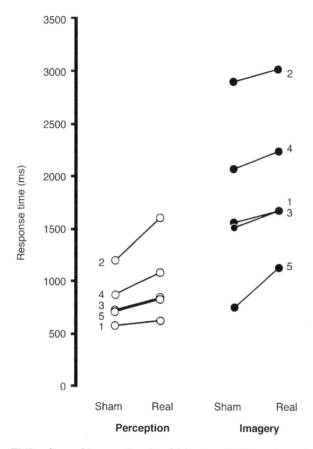

Figure 6.3   TMS and mental imagery. Results of delivering rTMS over the occipital cortex before perception and imagery conditions. "Real" TMS occurred when the magnetic field was directed into area 17, and sham rTMS occurred when the field was diverted away from the head. TMS over the visual cortex slowed response times in both perception and imagery conditions in all five subjects. (From Kosslyn et al., 1999, with permission.)

cortex may not be the same for tactile perception as for visual perception (see Zangaladze et al., 1999). If an area is involved in two tasks, but one of them requires involvement of, say, only 10% of that area's capacity, whereas the other demands, say, 70%, then the time window of compensation for each task may differ, and the task requiring 70% is far more likely to be affected by stimulation values intended to decrease activity in that area.

INTENTION AND ATTENTION

Studies of single-unit activity in the parietal cortex of monkeys have shown that orienting attention is closely associated with preparation of oculomotor responses. This result has led to the proposal that the role of the parietal cortex is best described as intentional (to emphasize the motor role) rather than attentional (Rizzolati, Fogassi, and Gallese, 1997; Snyder, Batista, and Andersen, 1997). To address this attention/intention debate, Rushworth, Ellison, and Walsh (2001) investigated the possibility that other attentional mechanisms might be tied to a particular response modality. In monkeys, the posterior region of the parietal cortex (area 7a) is anatomically connected to visual areas and the frontal eye fields (Goldman Rakic, 1998; Paus et al., 1997), whereas another region (area 7b) is connected with somatosensory and motor cortices (Goldman Rakic, 1998). It is significant that the two areas (7a and 7b) are not directly connected to each other (Cavada and Goldman-Rakic, 1993). The human homologues of the macaque areas are the PPC (area 7a) and the supramarginal gyrus (SMG, area 7b). On the basis of the anatomical connectivity of the SMG, Rushworth et al. hypothesized that rTMS applied here should interfere with motor attention but not with visual-orienting attention, whereas rTMS to the PPC should have the opposite pattern of effects. Figure 6.4 shows the task presented to subjects to test this.

The visual-orienting task did not require any motor decision component, simply a reflex response when the target red square was detected. Subjects fixated the center of the screen and were presented with a green rectangle, which cued the location at which the target red square would appear. Usually the cue correctly indicated the location of the target, but in 20% of trials the cue was invalid

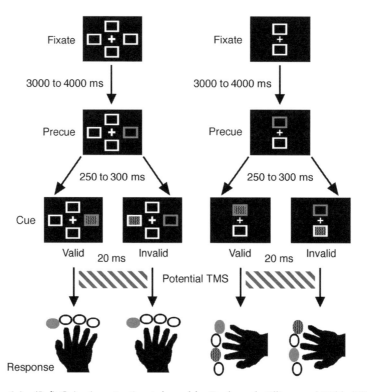

Figure 6.4 (*Left*) Orienting-attention task used by Rushworth, Ellison, and Walsh (2001). Subjects maintained fixation of a central cross between four white outline boxes (*first display at top*). The box outline changing from white to green (*second display*) was the precue that instructed subjects to orient to one of the four locations. After a gap of 250 or 350 msec, a target (a box center turning red) appeared at one of the four locations (*third display*). On 75% of trials, the precue was valid, and subjects correctly predicted the target position. On 20% of trials, the precue was invalid, and the target appeared in the box on the opposite side of fixation. On 5% of trials, no target was presented. The type of response made by the subjects is shown at the bottom of the figure. Each trial began once the subject was not pressing any of the four response keys. Whenever a target was presented at any of the four locations, subjects made the same key press response with the index finger. On the 5% of trials in which no target was presented, the subjects had to refrain from pressing the button for 2,000 msec. In 50% of invalidly cued trials and 10% of the more frequent validly cued trials, rTMS trains were delivered at random. (*Right*) Motor-attention task used by Rushworth, Ellison, and Walsh. Subjects fixated a central cross between two white boxes (*first display at top*). In this task, the box

and incorrectly cued the location. This is a version of the task Posner et al. (1984) used to show that patients with right parietal damage were impaired at switching attention from a cued to an uncued location. In the motor-attention task, the subjects were cued not for a visual location but for which finger to press in response to the onset of the target. Again, the cue was usually correct but was invalid on 20% of trials. This is a motor analogue of the visual-orienting response. Repetitive-pulse TMS (10 Hz for 500 msec) was applied over the right or left PPC or over the right or left SMG 20 msec after the onset of the target. The outcome showed that the two regions of parietal cortex are critical for motor intention (SMG) and visual attention (PPC). When rTMS was applied over the right PPC, there was an increase in reaction time on the invalid trials of the visual-orienting task (figure 6.5) but no effect on the motor-attention task (figure 6.6). When rTMS was applied over the left SMG, there was an increase in reaction time in the invalid trials of the motor-attention task for left-hand (figure 6.6a) and right-hand responses (figure 6.6b) but not in the visual-orienting task (figure 6.5). The physiological data from nonhuman primates, therefore, is consistent with respect to visual and motor attention, but whereas in the monkey the two functions require the intraparietal sulcus, in humans they have become lateralized, presumably reflecting the left hemisphere's crucial role in movement selection and execution and the right hemisphere's preeminence in visuospatial function.

---

centers were above and below fixation. At the beginning of each trial, the subject used the middle and index fingers of the same hand to press down the central two keys of the keypad (middle-finger home button and index-finger home button). The box outline turning from white to green (*second display*) was the cue that allowed subjects to direct motor attention to the response they would make in the final part of the trial (*third display*), 450 or 800 msec later when a target appeared in one of the boxes. Subjects responded to a lower target (*right*) by using the index finger to press the lowest key while simultaneously keeping the middle finger pressed on its home key at the center. The response to an upper target (*left*) was to press the middle finger on the upper key (top target) while simultaneously keeping the index finger on its home key at the center. In 80% of the trials, the cue was valid and correctly warned the subject which response would be made. The cue was invalid in 20% of trials. In 50% of invalidly cued trials and 10% of validly cued trials, rTMS trains were delivered at random. (After Rushworth, Ellison, and Walsh, 2001.)

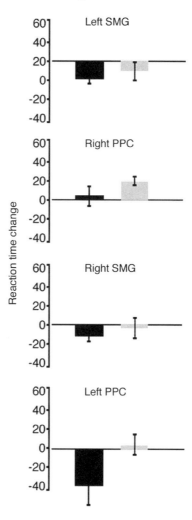

Figure 6.5 Orienting attention. Reaction time changes in valid (dark bars) and invalid (light bars) trials are shown depending on the site of rTMS application (left or right supra-marginal gyrus, SMG, or angular gyrus, PPC). Stimulation at any site on valid trials has mildly facilitatory or no effects. Stimulation over right PPC on invalid trials causes a significant reaction time increase.

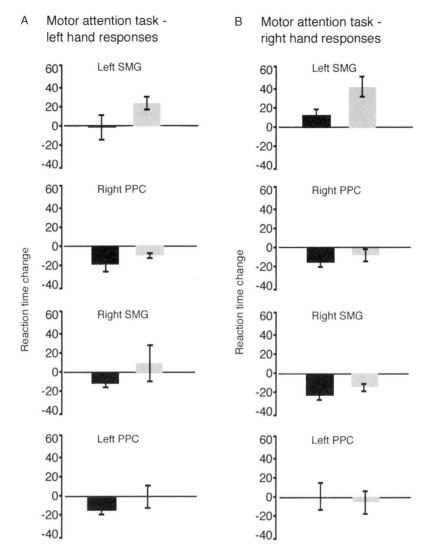

A   Motor attention task -
    left hand responses

B   Motor attention task -
    right hand responses

Figure 6.6   Motor-attention experiment results. The results for subjects using their left hand (*a*) or right hand (*b*) are shown separately. In general, rTMS at most sites has little effect or causes some facilitation. There was, however, a significant impairment when rTMS was delivered over the left SMG. The effect of rTMS over the left SMG was significantly greater on invalid trials (light bars), and reaction time was significantly slowed on invalid trials, regardless of whether the right (255 msec effect) or left (131 msec) hand was used.

COUNTING THE COST: MODELING ACALCULIA

The consequences of damage to the left or right parietal cortex are not always overtly visuospatial, attentional, or motoric in nature. Damage to the left parietal cortex can result in dyscalculia (acalculia), in which the patient appears to have lost the ability to conceptualize or use numbers any larger than around 4 (Dehaene, 1997; Butterworth, 1999). Recent neuroimaging work (Dehaene et al., 1996; Chochon et al., 1999; Cowell et al., 2000; Presenti et al., 2000; Stanescu-Cosson et al., 2000) consistently reveals the involvement of left and right parietal cortices in a range of numerical tasks, even though right parietal damage rarely has any effect on number ability. The few imaging studies of basic numerical processes such as enumerating dot arrays (Sathian et al., 1999; Piazza et al., in press) suggest that enumerating arrays of up to nine dots involves occipital lobes bilaterally and the right superior parietal lobule, which is consistent with patient studies showing right-hemisphere involvement in dot enumeration (Warrington and James, 1967; Warrington, 1982). So, although it is left-hemisphere-damaged patients who have difficulty manipulating numbers, the right hemisphere is clearly important in some basic numerical processing. Two alternative ways of thinking about numerical representation and manipulation are the "number line" and what one might call the "finger-counting" model. The number line account (Moyer and Bayer, 1976) conceptualizes numerical representation as a spatially represented continuum, which relies on the same mechanisms as other spatial abilities and therefore emphasizes the role of the right parietal cortex. The "finger-counting" model (Butterworth, 1999) emphasizes the role of the left parietal lobe as well as the coincidence of numerical deficits and Gerstmann's syndrome. To compare the respective roles of the two hemispheres, Göbel, Walsh, and Rushworth (2001) applied rTMS to the left or right parietal cortex unilaterally while subjects carried out a number estimation task. Subjects were given the number 65 as a standard, were presented with numbers between 31 and 99, and were asked to judge whether the number presented was larger or smaller than the standard. Repetitive-pulse TMS (500 msec, 10 Hz, 50–80% of stimulator output) was delivered at the onset of some of the numbers. As figure 6.7 shows, subjects displayed a normal "distance effect" on non-TMS

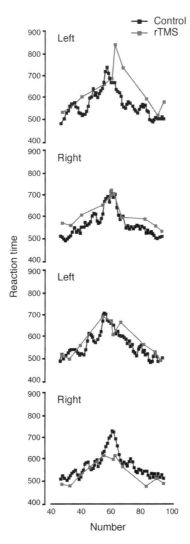

Figure 6.7   TMS effects on the mental number line. Stimulation over the PPC (*top two panels*) reveals a distinct slowing of responses for the left PPC when the numbers being compared are larger than the standard. Stimulation over the SMG (*bottom two panels*) had no systematic effects on subjects' ability to compare numbers or on the distribution of the judgments. (After Göbel et al., 2001.)

trials (i.e., the greater the difference between the standard number, 65, and the number presented, the shorter the reaction time to make the judgment). TMS over either left or right PPC increased reaction times, but TMS over neither the left nor the right SMG had any effect. The effect of left parietal stimulation only elevated reaction times for numbers larger than 65, and right parietal TMS elevated reaction times for most numbers. One immediately tempting explanation is that numerical representation is indeed spatial, and, as with visual space, the right hemisphere is important for both sides of space, whereas the left is involved in orienting and acting only in the right side of space (Mesulam, 1981). The problem for this explanation is that in vision it is damage to the right hemisphere that is more likely to cause visuospatial deficits, whereas damage to the left hemisphere is more likely to disrupt numerical abilities. An alternative explanation is that the "specter of compensation" (Lomber, 1999) underlies the neuropsychological findings: To wit, numerical judgments in intact individuals are a bilateral function of left and right parietal regions. In the absence of the right parietal cortex, the left parietal can recover function sufficiently to represent number with a diminished visuospatial system, perhaps due to disinhibition of the left PPC. In the absence of the left parietal cortex, however, the visuospatial mechanisms alone are insufficient for number comparison. Not all numerical abilities are disrupted by left parietal TMS, and the Number Stroop effect appears to be unaffected by TMS to the same sites that disrupt the number line (Göbel, personal communication). This finding is consistent with imaging data that show that anterior regions such as the cingulate cortex are more critical than posterior sites for dealing with the ambiguous information in Stroop (Pardo et al., 1990).

PERCEPTUAL LEARNING

So far we have concentrated on replicating the effects of brain lesions, on exploring differences between real and virtual lesions, or on the temporal aspects of TMS (chapter 5) as examples of how TMS can go beyond the neuropsychological data. There are, however, at least two other important conceptual areas that are a special province of TMS and into which classical neuropsychology usually can offer nothing or at best an occasional, fortuitous insight. These areas are learning and facilitations. A psychologist usually runs an experiment something like this: Take naive subjects, who may or may not have experienced the pleasure of being in an experiment before, then ask them to carry out an apparently trivial task such as detecting red vertical lines, saccading to or away from dots, reading nonsense words, or guessing whether something they didn't see was moving or stationary. As they do these tasks, for reasons they haven't been given, their performance is measured in reaction times and errors, and their brain activity is measured with PET, fMRI, MEG, or EEG or is disrupted by TMS. Thus, the literature contains a great deal of information about how bemused subjects do strange things in a dark room for the first time in their lives. Lives are seldom so exciting, and most people most of the time carry out their lives in familiar environments (airports), doing familiar things (searching for someone they met at the conference they just attended so they can avoid them) that they have done a thousand times before. A crucial task for cognitive neuroscience in the twenty-first century is to account for how the brain does such *routine* functioning: How does the brain do things that we are good at and with which we are familiar? Training patients to learn tasks so that one can assess the brain regions involved in a task when it is novel versus when it is trained compounds the problem of inference: patients are likely not only to be slow but also to learn the task by a different neural circuitry than normal subjects. Several TMS studies have now looked at the involvement of brain regions both when a task is novel and when it is familiar.

There seems to be little doubt that the PPC is important for conjunction visual search (chapter 5), but one can reasonably question whether the parietal cortex plays a role in all serial searches or whether it is only a critical part of the circuitry for searching in novel environments (such as being a naive subject in a novel laboratory experiment) but not for searching for familiar items in familiar environments. Walsh, Ashbridge, and Cowey (1998a) trained subjects on a visual search task until they could perform a previously inefficient visual search more efficiently. TMS was then applied to the parietal area and, despite the fact that TMS had disrupted performance when the task was novel and difficult, there was now no effect of stimulation (figure 6.8). Giving the same subjects a new

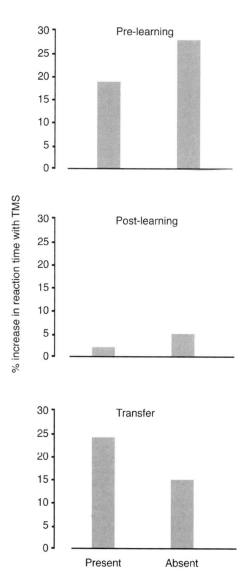

Figure 6.8 Changes in the role of the parietal cortex in visual search as a function of practice. When subjects are naive to a task, application of TMS over the right PPC increases the time taken to make the response, irrespective of whether the target is present or absent (*top*). Following a period of training TMS over the same site had no effect on reaction times (*middle*). Giving the subjects a new visual search task and applying TMS again over the right PPC reinstates the deficit in reaction time (*bottom*). (Replotted from Walsh, Ashbridge, and Cowey, 1998a.)

visual search task, to which learning did not transfer and thus produced a steep search function, reinstated the effects of TMS. Therefore, the preeminent role of the parietal cortex in visual search can be questioned. Perhaps it is necessary when searching for someone else's car keys but not for one's own because the latter is a very familiar task. By giving subjects a new visual search task after training, Walsh et al. presented subjects with two new variables—not only a new visual array, but also a new visuomotor association to be made between the new stimuli and the response. To explore this question, subjects again were presented with a novel visual search task, on which the naive subjects showed a steep reaction time × distractor slope (figure 6.9). At this stage, TMS over the right parietal cortex produced the expected deficit (figure 6.10). When subjects had learned the task over 1,500 trials, at which point they performed the search with a flat, parallel function (figure 6.9), TMS no longer disrupted the search function (figure 6.10). The subjects were then given the same visual search task but now were required to change the fingers with which they responded to the stimuli. Before and during training, subjects indicated a "target present" response with a key press by an index finger and a "target absent" response by a key press with a middle finger. This contingency was now reversed, and as figure 6.9 shows, subjects again reverted to a serial behavioral function, and the effect of TMS was reinstated (figure 6.10; Ellison, Rushworth, and Walsh, submitted). Thus, by exploiting the ability to use TMS at different stages of expertise, it has been shown that the right parietal cortex may have a role in search limited to new tasks, a role that is also at least partly visuomotor and not purely visuovisual.

Not all areas change their role so dramatically. Walsh et al. (1999) carried out a second learning experiment in which the effects of TMS over PPC and V5 were monitored as subjects learned a motion-form conjunction search. In this experiment, the essential role of the PPC in the search task was seen to diminish within 250 trials, after which TMS over PPC did not elevate reaction times on the search task, but V5 continued to be essential, and performance continued to be disrupted by TMS over this region (figure 6.11). This finding extends the learning data reported previously by Walsh, Ashbridge, and

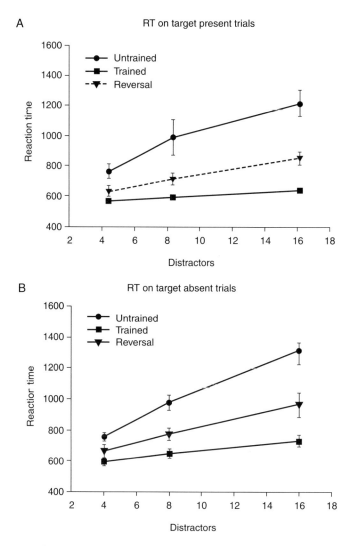

Figure 6.9   Behavioral performance of subjects on a conjunction visual search task for "target present" (*a*) and "target absent" (*b*) responses when the subjects are naive to the task (*top line in each graph*), following a period of training (*bottom line in each graph*), and when the same visual search task is presented but the subjects are required to change the finger with which they respond (*middle line in each graph*). The corresponding effects of TMS are shown in figure 6.10.

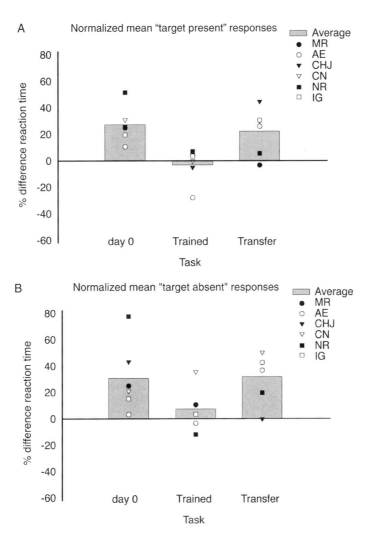

Figure 6.10 Changes in the visuomotor role of the PPC in a visual search task as a function of practice. As in the experiment shown in figure 6.8, TMS over the right PPC before learning slowed the subjects' responses (*left bar in each graph*), but there was no effect following a period of training (*middle bar in each graph*). When subjects were required to switch the fingers with which they responded, the effects of TMS were reinstated despite there being no change in the visual components of the task. (*a*) "Target present" responses, (*b*) "target absent" responses. Data are for search arrays with a single set size of 8 stimuli.

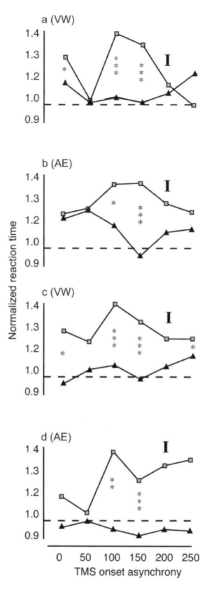

Figure 6.11   Learning a visual search task that is a conjunction of form and motion. There are no effects of TMS on the parietal cortex after 250 trials, suggesting that the role of the parietal cortex (TMS over the parietal cortex indicated by filled triangles) is diminished after an initial stimulus-response mapping is achieved. The top two graphs (*a*, *b*) show the effects of TMS on target present trials: TMS over V5 (open squares) has the greatest effect at around 100–150 msec after stimulus onset. The lower two graphs (*c*, *d*) show data for "target absent" trials where the main effects of V5 stimulation are again at approximately 100–150 msec after stimulus onset but also show a longer "tail" than the effect on target present trials. (After Walsh et al., 1999, with permission.)

Cowey (1998) and adds weight to the suggestion that PPC plays a critical role in forming new visuomotor response associations rather than solely in guiding visual binding of the different feature elements in an array.

TMS also can be used to affect the process of learning. Pascual-Leone et al. (1999) applied TMS to motor regions to enhance or impede selectively the degree of learning in an implicit motor-learning task. This use indicates that areas that are at a low level of a particular processing hierarchy (in this case the motor system) may be a substrate for learning. Pascual-Leone and colleagues specifically found that 1 Hz stimulation had a deleterious effect on learning, whereas 10 Hz stimulation had a positive effect (Tarazona et al., 1997; Pascual-Leone et al., 1999). A visual analogue of this experiment would reveal whether or not V5 is a candidate substrate of visual learning.

PERCEPTUAL MEMORY: A NEW WINDOW FOR TMS AND PSYCHOPHYSICS

Many events of interest occur not during or immediately after the presentation of stimuli but in between the responses to one event and the beginning of another, when the brain is making some sort of sense, perhaps, of what has just occurred in order to apply new probabilities to subsequent events (something the brain can do to our cost as well as to our advantage; see Wolford, Miller, and Gazzaniga, 2000). The most widely investigated of these phenomena is *priming* (the beginnings of memory). One theoretical framework (Tulving and Schacter, 1990) proposes that priming of physical attributes depends on a perceptual representation system (PRS) that is preconceptual and widely distributed. This proposal is supported by a body of psychophysical work indicating that perceptual memory (of which priming is a component) of the basic attributes of a visual scene (color, motion, orientation, and so on) is subserved by low-level mechanisms of perception, located beyond V1 but prior to regions involved in visual object perception (S. Magnussen, 2000; Magnussen and Greenlee, 1999). Also consistent with this work are neuropsychological patients, with posterior cortex lesions, who have impaired perceptual priming while maintaining relatively intact conceptual priming (Carlesimo et al., 1994; Gabrieli et al., 1995). Some neuropsychological and imaging studies, however, indicate that priming of visual attributes depends on the parietal cortex rather than on the functionally specialized regions of the extrastriate cortex (Farah et al., 1993; Marangolo et al., 1998). These accounts suggest that the parietal cortex either holds a representation of the stimulus or in some way biases the feature codes of the attributes, although the mechanisms of such biasing have not been elucidated.

It is difficult to test the role of brain areas in priming in neuropsychological studies of patients because patients are often much slower and more variable than controls, and damage to the sensory areas that process the visual elements also can cause impairments across a wide range of visual functions. Further, as we have argued in detail elsewhere (Walsh and Cowey, 1998; Pascual-Leone et al., 1999; Walsh and Rushworth, 1999), testing patients with long-standing lesions may tell us more about how the abnormal and readjusted brain operates than about how the normal brain works. To examine the perceptual memory and PRS hypotheses, Campana, Cowey, and Walsh (2002) used rTMS to disrupt briefly the visual processing in the striate, V5/MT, and parietal cortices during the intertrial interval of a motion discrimination task (figure 6.12). The intention was to interfere with the intertrial storage of the previously presented direction of motion while leaving discrimination accuracy unaffected. Subjects were given short trains of rTMS over the posterior occipital cortex, the extrastriate area V5/MT, or the right PPC while performing a visual motion direction discrimination task. A strong priming effect was observed in a control condition, which was abolished when area V5/MT was stimulated but not affected when magnetic stimulation was delivered over the striate or parietal sites (figure 6.13). The effect was specific both to stimulation site (TMS over V5 but not over the PPC or V1 disrupted motion priming) and to task (color priming was unaffected by TMS over V5; figure 6.14). The conclusion to be drawn here is that priming of visual motion seems to depend on the motion-sensitive sensory cortex rather than on control from the parietal cortex. The results parallel, in the motion domain, recent demonstrations of the importance of macaque areas V4 and TEO for priming in the colour and form domains (Bar and Biederman, 1999; Walsh et al., 2000) and also parallel Bisley and Pasternak's (2000) work on the effects of V5/MT lesions in macaque monkeys,

———

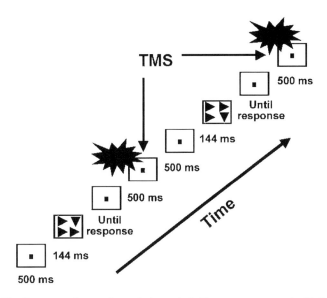

Figure 6.12   Sequence of events in a priming task. Subjects were presented with four panels of 100% coherent motion and required to detect the odd one out. TMS was applied in the 1,000 msec intertrial interval after subjects had made a response to the previous trial. The intention was to disrupt the representation of the previously detected direction of movement and to remove behavioral priming effects as a result. The same rationale was used to test color priming.

which has shown this sensory area to have a role to play in working memory for moving stimuli.

In addition to its intrinsic interest, this experiment is so far the only example of TMS used within the framework of perceptual memory (Magnussen, 2000; Magnussen and Greenlee, 1999; Magnussen, 2000), which opens up many possibilities for probing psychophysical functions with TMS, something that has proved difficult to achieve so far (see Miller et al., 1996; Corthout et al., 1999a,b; Kammer, 1999, for exceptions) as a result of the spatial and temporal overlap of processing in striate cortex. With the use of delayed responses, however, TMS can be applied to disrupt psychophysical functions at different stages of encoding, storage, and recall. This rich vein of possibilities is especially amenable to TMS because the psychophysical foundations have been laid already.

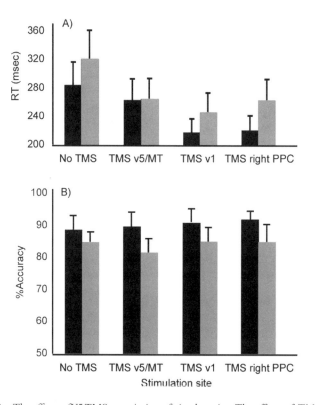

Figure 6.13   The effects of V5 TMS on priming of visual motion. The effects of TMS on motion priming are specific to the site of stimulation. (*A*) Reaction times as a function of SAME/DIFFERENT trials (dark/light bars respectively) and TMS site. The first pair of histograms (No TMS) shows a priming effect (SAME faster than DIFFERENT: mean reaction times (S.E.) in msec, 284 (32) and 319 (40) respectively), so too the third (TMS V1) and fourth (TMS right PPC) pair, which show reaction times for trials when TMS was applied over the striate or parietal cortex. The priming effect in these trials was maintained; mean reaction times (S.E.) in msec: TMS over V1, SAME trials, 220 (18); DIFFERENT trials, 247 (27); TMS over PPC, SAME trials, 222 (19); DIFFERENT trials, 262 (29). As the second pair of histograms shows (TMS V5/MT), there is no priming effect when V5/MT was the targeted region of TMS: SAME trials 264 (28), DIFFERENT trials 265 (28). (*B*) Accuracy data as a function of SAME/DIFFERENT trials. (After Campana, Cowey, and Walsh, 2002.)

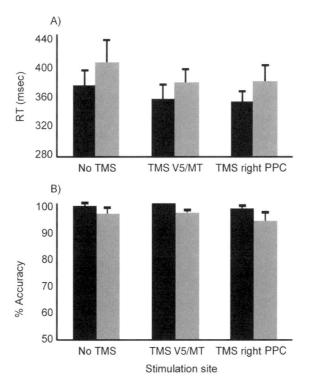

Figure 6.14   The effects of V5 TMS on color priming. The effects of V5 stimulation on motion priming are specific to motion. (*A*) Reaction times as a function of SAME/DIFFERENT trials and TMS site. The priming effect (SAME faster than DIFFERENT) is seen in the baseline condition; mean reaction times (S.E.) in msec: SAME trials 379(9), DIFFERENT 409 (14). This behavioral pattern is unaffected by either V5 or right parietal cortex stimulation. V5 TMS mean reaction times (S.E.): SAME trials, 360 (9), DIFFERENT trials 381 (8); PPC TMS mean reaction times (S.E.): SAME trials 356 (6), DIFFERENT trials 383 (10). (*B*) Accuracy data as a function of SAME/DIFFERENT trials.

Paradoxical Functional Facilitations

Damage to the human brain can have a variety of debilitating effects on the sufferer, and the range of disabilities is the raw material of neuropsychology. Curiously, brain damage occasionally can result in an improvement of function or a return of a previously compromised ability. The most famous example is the original Sprague effect. Sprague (1966) removed regions of the right occipitotemporal cortex and produced a corresponding hemianopia in the contralateral visual field. By subsequently lesioning the left superior colliculus, Sprague was able to restore responses to visual stimuli in the left visual field and concluded that the original deficit was due to inhibition or suppression of the right colliculus by the left.

There are now many replications and reports of similar effects in the animal literature and several reports of paradoxical functional facilitation[4] in human subjects (see Kapur, 1996). The two main classes of facilitation have been termed *restorative,* wherein a hitherto deficient function has returned (as in the Sprague effect), and *enhancing,* in which some damage or loss of function results in patients performing better than normal subjects at some task. Both classes of facilitation reveal much of interest about the dynamic interactions between different modalities or even components of sensory modalities. Nevertheless, as Kapur notes, "such findings have often been ignored or undervalued in the brain-behavior research literature" (1996). Perhaps this is because paradoxical facilitations are less common and less salient than deficits and also more difficult to interpret. Recent neurocomputing work may be useful in imposing some direction as well as constraints on the search for and interpretation of facilitatory effects of TMS (Hilgetag, Kotter, and Young, 1999; Young, Hilgetag, and Scannell, 1999, 2000). One simulation, for example, showed that the connectivity of a cortical area was a strong predictor of the effects of lesions on the rest of the network as well as of how that area responded to a lesion elsewhere in the network. This may seem like a truism, but the kind of connectivity analysis

---

4. The term *paradoxical functional facilitations* is taken from Kapur's (1996) enlightening review of a neglected area in neurology and neuropsychology.

offered by these models is not really taken into account in classical lesion analysis (see also Robertson and Murre, 1999; Rossini and Pauri, 2000), and the modelling work has begun to make these predictions explicit and testable. Moreover, in the past, paradoxical facilitations could not be induced at will; hence, investigators depended on the serendipity of nature, a limitation that TMS promises to overcome.

Walsh et al. (1998b) stimulated visual area V5 in an attempt to model the "motion blind" patient L.M. (Zihl et al., 1983; McLeod et al., 1989), and indeed V5 stimulation did impair performance on visual search tasks that involved scanning complex motion displays. On displays in which motion was absent or irrelevant to task performance, subjects were faster with TMS than in control trials (figure 6.15). This result can be interpreted as evidence that the separate visual modalities may compete for resources, and the disruption of the motion system may have liberated other visual areas from its influence. Competition is readily accepted between stimuli within a receptive field (e.g., Moran and Desimone, 1985; Desimone and Duncan, 1995) and also between hemispheres, but potential competition between areas within a hemisphere has received less attention. In this experiment, the subjects received blocks of trials of a single type and therefore knew whether the upcoming stimulus array would contain movement or color or form as the important parameter. When the types of trials were interleaved such that the subject did not have advance information, the enhancing effects of TMS were not obtained. Thus, it seems that a combination of priming (due to the advanced knowledge of the stimuli) and weakening of the V5 system (by TMS) were required to enhance performance on color and form tasks. Conceptually similar is the finding of Seyal, Ro, and Rafal (1995), who, as we saw in chapter 5, observed increases in tactile sensitivity as a result of stimulation of the somatosensory cortex ipsilateral to fingers being tested, and the interpretation in that study also is based on disinhibition of the unstimulated hemisphere.

As mentioned earlier, paradoxical functional facilitation can be restorative or enhancing. Studies on parietal function in attention provide elegant examples of the capability of TMS to induce both of these phenomena and possibly to

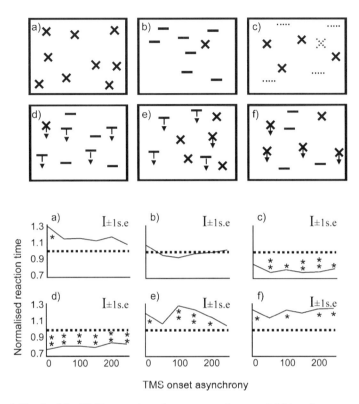

Figure 6.15   Applying TMS to a region of cortex can enhance or inhibit peformance on different tasks. The top panels show six visual search tasks in which subjects were required to detect the presence or absence of a target; the bottom panel shows the effects of applying TMS to area V5. In two tasks, (tasks *a* and *b*) there is little or no effect of TMS. When TMS is applied to V5 during a search requiring attention to motion (tasks *e* and *f*) performance is significantly slower with TMS. Tasks on which attention to attributes other than motion is required are faciliated by TMS over V5. Dotted line at 1 represents reaction times without TMS. Solid lines show reaction times with TMS relative to without. (From Walsh et al., 1998b, with permission.)

lend itself to therapeutic applications. Oliveri et al. (1999a) used TMS in a tactile stimulus–detection task to demonstrate that the right but not the left parietal cortex is critical for detection not only of contralateral but also of ipsilateral stimuli (see also "Adding Insult to Injury," chapter 8). They found that bimanual discrimination is disrupted more readily than unimanual tasks, but only during right (not left) parietal TMS. Most important, they showed that the contribution of the right parietal cortex takes place 40 msec after the tactile stimuli are applied, hence suggesting involvement of late cortical events. Olivieri et al. (1999b) then applied TMS to patients with right-hemisphere lesions. When stimuli were applied simultaneously to both hands, patients often failed to detect the stimulus on the left side. Stimulation (at intensities 10% higher than used in normal subjects) of the left frontal but not the parietal cortex significantly reduced the rate of extinction. Therefore, as in the animal model (Lomber and Payne, 1996), transient disruption of the healthy hemisphere restores spatial attention and improves neglect. These results support the notion of an interhemispheric competition (possibly asymmetrical) of cortical or subcortical structures to explain facilitations. Furthermore, they provide the first clear example of restorative paradoxical functional facilitation induced by TMS and suggest that such strategies might be applicable to speed up neurorehabilitation. The notion of interhemispheric competition in guiding attention was put to test directly by Hilgetag, Theoret, and Pascual-Leone (2001) using an "off-line" (or distal, see chapter 4) rTMS paradigm. They found ipsilateral enhancement of visual attention, compared to normal performance (figure 6.16), produced by rTMS of the parietal cortex at stimulation parameters known to reduce cortical excitability. Healthy, right-handed volunteers received rTMS (1 Hz, 10 min) over the right or left parietal cortex (at P3 and P4 EEG coordinate points, respectively). This type of stimulation is expected to disrupt cortical function transiently by inducing a depression of excitability that outlasts the duration of the rTMS train itself (Chen et al., 1997a; Maeda et al., 2000). Subsequently, the subjects' attention to ipsilateral visual targets improved significantly while contralateral attention diminished. Additionally, correct detection of bilateral stimuli decreased

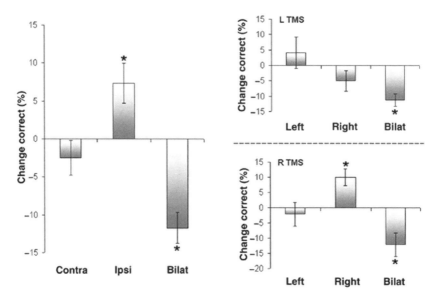

Figure 6.16   Changes in correct stimulus detection after rTMS over the parietal cortex. The diagrams are based on changes in the number of correctly detected stimuli (relative to the total number of presented stimuli) averaged for both stimulus sizes and all subjects. (*a*) The pooled data show a significant increase in performance ipsilateral to the parietal rTMS location (increase in relative percentage points by 7.3%, [SEM]: 2.6%), and a trend to decreased contra-lateral performance (reduction by 2.5%, SEM: 2.3%). In addition, detection of bilateral stimuli decreased significantly (−11.7%, SEM: 2.0%). These trends are also apparent after separating data for (*b*) left parietal TMS and (*c*) right parietal rTMS. Significant trends (as determined by z-tests) are marked by asterisks. (Modified from Hilgetag et al., 2001, with permission.)

significantly, coupled with an increase in erroneous responses for ipsilateral unilateral targets. Application of the same rTMS paradigm to motor cortex as well as sham magnetic stimulation indicated that the effect was specific for stimulation of the parietal cortex. These results underline the potential of focal brain dysfunction to produce behavioral improvement, and they provide experimental proof that TMS can be used for the induction of enhancing paradoxical functional facilitations.

Lost for Words: Studies of Language Processing

One of the most dramatic demonstrations of TMS is magnetically induced speech arrest, and several groups have now reported that rTMS over the left frontal or either the left or right motor cortex can cause subjects to cease speaking or to stutter or repeat segments of words. As far as the neuropsychologist is concerned, this work is very preliminary, no more than a calibration experiment, in fact, because the emphasis has been on localizing the site of stimulation or establishing the most reliable parameters for speech arrest or both.

Pascual-Leone et al. (1991c) were the first to induce speech arrest (25 Hz rTMS with a round coil) in a population of epileptic subjects awaiting surgery, and the TMS determination of the dominant hemisphere in all six subjects matched that obtained in the WADA test. The motivation for this and other early experiments on speech was the possibility that TMS could be used to replace the invasive WADA test. The results in this respect have been variable, largely because of the different hardware and criteria for arrest adopted by different groups. Following Pascual-Leone et al.'s demonstration, the effect was replicated, again in epileptic patients, by Jennum et al. (1994, at 30 Hz rTMS), whose data also showed a strong concordance with the results of the amylobarbital test. In studies that may require hundreds of trials, 25 and 30 Hz is too high a frequency, but a later study by Epstein and colleagues (1996), which attempted to identify optimum parameters for arrest, identified 4–8 Hz as the optimum range for arrest in normal subjects. However, Epstein et al. used an iron-core stimulation coil that may well have effects deeper in the brain than do standard coils. They also were able to distinguish between arrest associated with frontal cortex stimulation and in the absence of apparent effects on facial muscles and effects associated with loss of control of the facial muscles. There have been some attempts to examine language functions beyond demonstrations of speech arrest, but the best of these experiments have not tested a theoretical prediction and can really be considered as further examples of generalized speech effects. Flitman et al. (1998), for example, applied rTMS over frontal and parietal lobes while subjects judged whether a word was congruent with a simultaneously presented picture. With TMS, subjects were slower to verify the congruency, but it is not clear whether they were impaired on any particular cognitive aspect of this task or the load on the language system was greater than in the control condition of stating whether or not the word and picture were surrounded by a rectangular frame.

Recent studies (Epstein et al., 1999; Bartres-Faz et al., submitted; Stewart et al., 2001a) mark the end of this ten-year period of trying to ascertain the location and reliability of speech arrest effect in normal subjects. All three studies obtained speech arrest lateralized to the left hemisphere with frontal stimulation. Epstein et al. suggest that their effects are due to motor cortex stimulation, but this suggestion is difficult to reconcile with the left unilateral dominance of the effects and also with Stewart et al., who provide independent anatomical and physiological evidence of a dissociation between frontal stimulation and pure motor effects. Both Bartres-Faz's and Stewart's studies locate the critical site of stimulation to be over the middle frontal gyrus, dorsal to the inferior frontal gyrus and what is usually referred to as Broca's area. These two studies are in agreement with lesion data (e.g., Rostomily et al., 1991), electrical stimulation mapping (Penfield and Roberts, 1959; Ojemann and Mateer, 1979; Ojemann, 1983), and PET studies (Ingvar, 1983)—all of which have shown several areas, including the middle temporal gyrus, to be important in speech production.

Speech arrest can be obtained from direct electrical stimulation of so many brain regions that it clearly will be very difficult to try to pin down a single area with TMS. The right strategy would seem to be to use TMS to produce language-related dissociations that address theoretical questions. This area is wide open for new approaches using TMS. Human lesions that produce language deficits are typically large; animal lesions, of course, cannot address the question of language. To make use of the localization of speech arrest sites, it is not necessary to induce such salient effects on every trial, and we anticipate that the typical neuropsychology experiment will be based on stimulation at intensity levels too low to induce arrest but sufficient to incur reaction-time costs in verbal tasks. Stewart et al. (2000) for example, have begun to probe parts of the language system by testing the predictions that BA37 has a role in phonological retrieval and object naming (Burnstine et al., 1990; Price, Wise, and Frackowiack, 1996; Moore and Price, 1999). Repetitive-pulse TMS was applied over the posterior region of BA37 of the left and right hemispheres and over the vertex. The rTMS had significant effects on picture naming but no effect on word reading, nonword reading, or color naming. Thus, with respect to object encoding and naming, the posterior region of BA37 would seem to be critical for recognition. Picture naming was also examined by Topper et al. (1998), who applied single-pulse TMS over Wernicke's area and motor cortex. Somewhat paradoxically, TMS over Wernicke's area for 500–1000 msec prior to picture presentation resulted in faster reaction times than those in control trials. The effect was specific to task and area, and Topper et al. concluded that TMS "is able to facilitate lexical processes due to a general preactivation of language-related neuronal networks when delivered over Wernicke's area." Although these effects are intriguing, they raise several questions about why single-pulse TMS would have facilitatory effects within a system (see chapter 4 for discussion of reaction-time decreases and the section "Paradoxical Functional Facilitations" in this chapter). If generalized arousal within the language system were a tenable explanation, one would have to predict similarly modulated gains whenever TMS was applied over a language-related area, which seems unlikely to be the case. More than in any other kind of result, it is important that the apparently facilitatory effects of TMS are grounded in theoretical frameworks and that the mechanisms proposed in one modality are applicable to others. If, for example, TMS over Wernicke's area facilitates picture naming, then similar facilitations should be obtainable in other modalities. It is also puzzling that lower-intensity TMS produced larger facilitation effects than higher-intensity TMS in this study. Further studies of these effects are clearly necessary, but perhaps before basing any further conclusions on a direct facilitation, one should await evidence that an area's primary function can be disabled by TMS.

Grafman et al. (1994) studied language-related memory function. Subjects received rTMS at 20 Hz, 120% of motor threshold for 500 msec, over one of several cortico-cortical sites while they were presented with a list of words. Their recall of the words was then tested, and selective deficits in recall were produced only by rTMS over left midtemporal or either left or right dorsolateral frontal cortex when the stimulation was applied either at the onset or with a delay of 250 msec after onset of the visual word display.

WHAT IS IN A VERB?

Studies in which neurolinguistic questions are addressed with TMS, rather than just the possibility of disrupting speech output, are beginning to be conducted. A recent study by Shapiro et al. (2001) used TMS to study grammatical distinctions in the frontal cortex and demonstrated the role of the left frontal cortex in representation of verbs as a grammatical class. Selective deficits in producing verbs relative to nouns in speech are well documented in neuropsychology and have been associated with left-hemisphere frontal cortical lesions resulting from a variety of causes. This functional-anatomical link, though problematic, has led some researchers to propose that verb retrieval is mediated by left frontal or frontostriatal circuits that also subserve motor planning. Previous attempts to verify the neural substrates of verb retrieval with data from unimpaired speakers have been inconclusive. Though electrophysiological studies have shown increased left-lateralized anterior positivity when verbs are produced compared to nouns, functional neuroimaging either has failed to reveal differences in patterns of activation between nouns and verbs or has shown that verb generation recruits a patchwork of areas in the left hemisphere (see Shapiro et al., 2001, for discussion). It is not obvious from these data whether frontal circuits are engaged necessarily and specifically in verb production.

Shapiro et al. (2001) used rTMS to target a portion of prefrontal cortex along the midfrontal gyrus anterior and superior to Broca's area while subjects performed a linguistic task involving regular nouns or verbs. The experiment was divided into four blocks, each of which consisted of two sets of eighty trials separated by an interval of 300 pulses of rTMS at 1 Hz and 110% of the motor threshold intensity, applied with a focal figure-of-eight coil. A 10 min rest period followed each block to allow the effects of rTMS to wash out. The first two blocks were control blocks in which the TMS coil was positioned to produce a sensation similar to real stimulation, but with no cortical interference. In each trial, the subject was presented with a stimulus word (either a noun or a verb) for 250 msec, followed for another 250 msec by a symbolic cue indicating the morphological form in which the word was to be produced aloud—singular

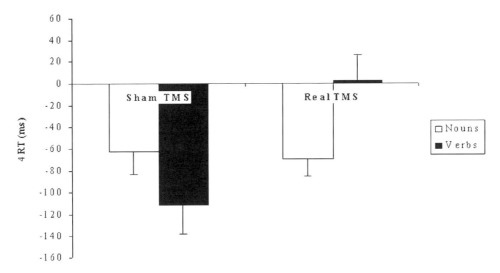

Figure 6.17   The bar histogram displays the effects of rTMS on production of pseudowords used as nouns and verbs. Statistically equivalent decreases in average response latency were observed after sham stimulation for both nouns and verbs. However, real rTMS to the left but not to the right frontal cortex led to a decrease in average response times for nouns (due to practice effect) following the rTMS, but no such decrease for verbs. Similar results were obtained when using real nouns and verbs rather than pseudowords used as nouns or verbs. Therefore, the results demonstrate a critical role for the left prefrontal cortex in processing verbs because disruption of function in this area prevented the expected practice-induced decrease in response times. (From Shapiro et al., 2001, with permission.)

($\diamond$) or plural ($\diamond\diamond\diamond$) for nouns (e.g., *song, songs*), third-person singular ($\triangle$) or plural ($\triangle\triangle\triangle$) for verbs (e.g., *sings, sing*). Plural and singular stimulus words were paired randomly with cues so that the required manipulation (if any) for each stimulus was unpredictable. It is important to note that given the task design, the manipulations were phonologically identical for nouns and verbs, involving addition and subtraction of the morpheme /s/. Nouns and verbs were presented in alternate blocks in an order that varied by subject.

Figure 6.17 summarizes the results. Following sham stimulation, average response latencies decreased markedly from baseline for both nouns and verbs.

The magnitude of this decrease did not differ significantly between word classes, and there was no interaction between time and grammatical class. When real stimulation was applied, the results were strikingly different. There was again a decrease in average response time for nouns, identical to the decrease in the sham condition. However, average response time for verbs *increased* following rTMS, a change that was both qualitatively and quantitatively different from the change seen after sham stimulation and that suggests that verb production specifically had been hindered.

Word production is a multistage process with separate components involved in the computation of a word's meaning, grammatical function, and sound structure; nouns and verbs may differ prototypically in any or all of these dimensions. Shapiro et al.'s results demonstrate for the first time that neural circuits in the left frontal cortex adjacent to Broca's area are critical at some stage in the spoken production of verbs by unimpaired individuals and illustrate the potential of TMS in studies of linguistic processing.

The Self-Engineering Brain

A "Chaos of Being"

It is revealing of the way in which cognitive neuroscience is constructed that the study of plasticity has become a field in its own right. We already have discussed the problems of assuming chronometric linearity in cognitive functions (see "Chronometric Impossibilities," chapter 5), and we also have seen that brain areas can change their role as a function of practice (chapter 6). But the problems go deeper. The idea that we can arrest brain function at some particular point in a stream carries the assumption that we already know something about that stream, already know in fact where the brain is up to in a certain chain of events. This assumption has to be made, of course, in order to carry out any kind of temporally based experiment at all, and we have to live with the consequences and limitations (see "Perceptual Learning," chapter 6), but it is humbling to reconsider those limitations. Let us begin with the fact that the brain is never at rest and never switches off at the start of an experiment simply to enable the neuroscientist to begin with a clean slate. Let's add the assumption that we cannot be sure of what the initial state of the brain happens to be in any given experiment—we hope no one would disagree. We could just shrug off these problems and get on with tractable experiments, but a third fact compounds the problem: The brain is likely to be in two different states when it performs the same act under the same experimental conditions twice in succession. That this is so can be seen in the effects of priming, for example, of even simple sensory stimuli ("Perceptual Memory," chapter 6). Thomas Carlyle aptly captured the problem (albeit in a different context): "*actual events are nowise so simply related to each other as parent and offspring are: every single event is the offspring not of one but of all other events, prior or contemporaneous, and will in its turn combine with all others to give birth to new: . . . it is an ever working* Chaos of Being." And in that chaos we are forever trying to hit a moving target, be it a sensory decision, a visuomotor transformation, a reward signal, awareness, or an action plan. Studies of plasticity are concentrated on understanding recovery from injury or the effects of acquiring expertise, but plasticity is not a special state of the nervous system—*plasticity is the normal state of the nervous system*. A full, coherent account of any sensory or cognitive function will build into its framework the ongoing changes that occur as the brain continuously learns from and updates its model of the world. The evidence for this view is overwhelming: adaptation in the short and long term, priming, order effects in experiments, the effects of feedback in experiments, and the response of subjects and cerebral hemispheres to changing probability frequencies (Wolford, Miller, and Gazzaniga, 2000). Crick and Koch (1998) sum up the problem in the context of consciousness of a single event: "There, has . . . to be a way of imposing a *temporary unity* on the activities of all the neurons that are relevant at that moment" (our italics). True—and the probability of any two moments of temporary unity being the same is close to nil. This is not a counsel of despair; that would be to suggest that one should ignore the problem. The solution in psychology is twofold: one can design experiments that as far as possible negate the small changes that may occur in brain circuits over the course of experiments, a hugely successful strategy as the current state of cognitive neuroscience testifies; or one can try to understand plasticity *in the context of normal behavior*—a virtually untouched question. So far in this book we have concentrated on the former approach, but TMS also may provide a way to begin thinking about the normal state of plasticity of the active brain. Because the study of plasticity is a separate discipline, TMS studies have been concerned with development, recovery from injury and learning, but the application of

TMS in these areas suggests ways in which experiments on the moment-to-moment plasticity may be approached.

The necessity of understanding change also has touched studies using MRI. One must assume that the brain is in a stable cognitive state during the experimental task and in the baseline condition. Grabowski and Damasio (2000) have discussed at length the problems inherent in this and other assumptions, and much of their analysis applies to TMS. Poldrack (2000) also has discussed the problems of imaging plasticity and raises a similar set of questions: How does one assess the impact of improvements in performance, the differences between baseline states in two different experimental sessions, and possible changes in functional connectivity between areas? Studies using TMS can bypass the problem of interpreting the meaning of correlations between changes in brain activation and behavioral performance, but the theoretical questions themselves remain. Subjects will no more "empty their minds" for TMS experiments than for any other kind of procedure. If we are to reverse engineer the brain successfully, we must be mindful of the fact that it is constantly reengineering itself.

IN CAJAL'S FOOTSTEPS . . . AGAIN

We have seen that TMS can be used to investigate the way in which the relative contributions of an area to a task can change as a function of explicit learning ("Perceptual Learning," chapter 6). Other changes in neuronal circuits can occur for many different reasons throughout life—as a function of normal development, as a response to acute or chronic injury or to implicit learning, or even as a result of TMS targeted at the appropriate brain regions and tasks. Adaptation to congenital illness, such as blindness, also may be considered as evidence of the malleability of neuronal circuits (Cohen et al., 1997). Magnetic stimulation can be used to probe all of these levels of plasticity, from changes in the range of seconds to those that occur over years of normal development or rehabilitation. Most of the studies using TMS to investigate plasticity have been carried out in the sensory and motor cortex, but the paradigms used clearly have applications in cognitive experiments and have yet to be exploited to their full potential.

The idea that the adult brain is capable of plasticity is not new, nor is the idea that the mechanisms of plasticity may be either a strengthening of old connections or a development of new ones. Ramón y Cajal made the point with reference to skill acquisition:

> the work of a pianist, speaker, mathematician, thinker etc., is inaccessible for the untrained human, as the acquisition of new abilities requires many years of mental and physical practice. In order to fully understand this complicated phenomenon, it is necessary to admit, in addition to the strengthening of pre-established organic pathways, the establishment of new ones, through ramification and progressive growth of dendritic arborizations and nervous terminals. . . . Such development takes place in response to exercise, while it stops and may be reversed in brain spheres that are not cultivated. (1904)

In addition to the ever-present plasticity, different kinds of changes in organization occur in several different time windows—years and months, weeks and days, minutes—and TMS has been used to look through all of these windows.

BABES AND ARMS

The development of motor coordination continues throughout childhood and into adolescence, and one of the problems the nervous system has to solve is how to maintain motor control over a period of life during which an individual may grow from 0.5 to 2 m and during which the rate of that growth may vary over a twentyfold range (Tanner, Whitehouse, and Takaishi, 1966; Eyre, Miller, and Ramesh, 1991). Not only is the child growing in height, but the limbs are growing, and the area swept by any movement changes as a result. One proposed solution to the engineering problem of keeping timing of movements stable is that the nervous system employs constant conduction times rather than a more complex mechanism that would be able to track changing timing requirements throughout development (Dorf, 1986). Eyre, Miller, and Ramesh (1991) tested this possibility directly by measuring conduction times and sensitivity to TMS (in the form of EMG threshold) in more than four hundred subjects between the ages of thirty-two weeks and fifty-two years. They applied TMS over the motor cortex and the cervical spine and recorded EMG from the biceps and the hypothenar muscles. Figure 7.1 shows clear results: cortical-evoked EMGs decreased in latency from thirty-two weeks until approximately two years of age and then plateaud at adult levels (figure 7.1C–F). The latency of responses following cervical stimulation were relatively constant until four to five years of age and thereafter increased in proportion to arm length across all ages. The sensitivity of the motor cortex to TMS (the motor threshold) also decreased markedly over time, but unlike the characteristic of the delay changes, the output of the TMS pulse required to elicit an EMG response continued to decrease until approximately sixteen years of age (figure 7.1G). In comparison, the peripheral sensitivity to TMS, undergoes a less-dramatic change but also plateaus at approximately five years of age (figure 7.1H).

An analogue of Eyre, Miller, and Ramesh's study was carried out in infant and adult macaque monkeys by Flament et al. (1992). The latency of motor-evoked responses reached adult ranges between four and six months of age, and there was a clear increase in sensitivity to TMS between six and eight months, after which the threshold for MEPs reached a plateau (figure 7.2). These time windows of change corresponded with the onset of behavioral change in the form of the acquisition of full-precision finger movements in the macaques (Lawrence and Kuypers, 1968; Lawrence and Hopkins, 1976), which are used for the retrieval of food and also for grooming, a behavior that also begins to occur at approximately six months (Hinde, Rowell, and Spencer-Booth, 1964).

Neither the Eyre, Miller, and Ramesh study nor the Flament et al. study is intended to approach a question of cognition, but their longitudinal nature and the clear link they establish between brain development and behavior are strong examples of the way in which TMS can be used in longitudinal studies. A simple example of how this methodology might be extended to psychology is in developmental dyslexia. Some authors, for example, have emphasized the role of the motor system as an example of deficits in processing fast temporal information.

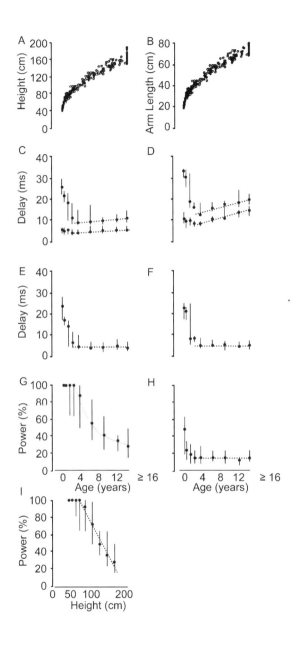

It is clear from Eyre, Miller, and Ramesh's data that some critical changes in peripheral motor processes occur from the age of five (figure 7.1B), whereas more central processes peak at around two years with respect to latency (figure 7.1E) but change throughout adolescence with respect to sensitivity (figure 7.1G). It would be a strong test of this approach to dyslexia to see if central motor development can be associated with difficulties in learning to read or in developing other skills that correlate with reading problems (see also Heinen et al., 1998). Application in monkeys might go further and test the effects of lesions on development of central motor processes.

TMS also has been used to study plasticity over shorter time periods and with more direct cognitive goals, and these studies have taken one of three approaches. One approach is to use motor outputs to assess the extent of cortical reorganization following brain damage. This approach has been applied mainly to changes in motor maps following transient and reversible blocking of sensory input (Brasil-Neto et al., 1992b, 1993) or to patients who have undergone amputation (Cohen et al., 1991a; Kew et al., 1994; Pascual-Leone et al., 1996). The second approach is to use TMS in its virtual-lesion mode to assess the functional relevance of any supposed reorganization of function (Pascual-Leone and Torres, 1993; Pascual-Leone et al., 1995a, 1995; Cohen et al., 1997). The third approach has been to use TMS to influence plasticity (Pascual-Leone et al., 1996, 1999b; Stefan et al., 2000) or as a secondary technique when plasticity has

---

Figure 7.1 Developmental motor studies and TMS. Stimulus intensity and MEPs plotted according to age and height in subjects ranging from zero to fifty-five years ($n = 308$). (*A*) and (*B*) show height and arm length in relation to age. (*C*) and (*D*) show the conduction delays following TMS of the motor cortex (*upper curves*) and cervical spinal root (*lower curves*). MEPs were recorded from the biceps brachii (*C*) and hypothenar muscles (*D*). Central motor-conduction delay shown for activation of biceps brachii (*E*) and hypothenar muscles (*F*). (*G*) and (*H*) show the stimulus intensity required to evoke an MEP following TMS over the motor cortex (MEP, biceps) and the cervical spine (hypothenar MEP) (*I*) shows the intensity required to evoke an MEP as a function of height. The absciccae cut off at greater than sixteen years because values reach a lifetime plateau at this age. The values for each data point are medians. (From Eyre, Miller, and Ramesh, 1991, with permission.)

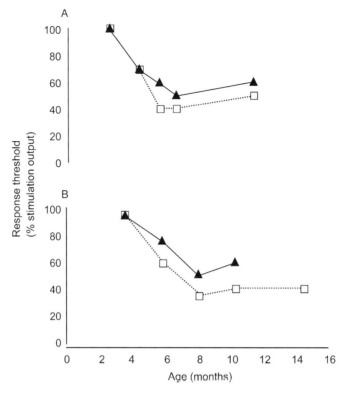

Figure 7.2   EMG thresholds plotted as function of age in two infant monkeys (*A* and *B*). Before five months, there is no difference between relaxed (*triangles*) and active (*squares*) motor thresholds. Beyond five months, increased spontaneous activity was correlated with 10–20% lower thresholds. (From Flament, Hall, and Lemon, 1992, with permission.)

been modulated by other means such as practice (Classen et al., 1998) or drugs (Bütefisch et al., 2000).

PHANTOM MAPS

The reorganization of pathways following injury can occur over a period of minutes. Brasil-Neto et al. (1992b) have used TMS as a secondary measure to

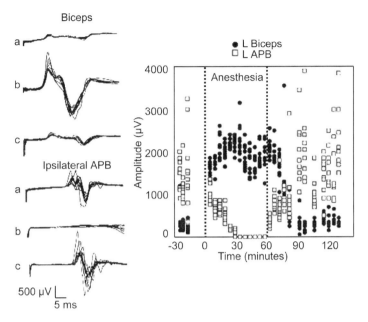

Figure 7.3 (*Left*) Ten superimposed MEPs from biceps and ipsilateral abductor pollicis bre-vis (APB) (*a*) before anesthesia, (*b*) during anaesthetic block, and (*c*) after anesthesia in one sub-ject. (*Right*) Amplitudes of MEPs from biceps and ipsilateral APB as a function of the time course of the experiment (same subject). (From Brasil-Neto et al., 1992b, with permission.)

investigate the time course of changes in the motor output system following deafferentation. Subjects received a nerve block and local anesthesia to deafferent the forearm and hand selectively and transiently, and TMS-elicited EMGs were recorded from the APB and the bicep (the muscles immediately proximal to the cuff and site of anesthesia) before, during, and after deafferentation. Within min-utes of the nerve block, MEPs recorded from the bicep began to increase in am-plitude, indicating a rapid unmasking of preexisting, but normally inhibited connections (figure 7.3). After anesthesia ended, the MEPs returned to normal over a period of approximately 20 min (see also Brasil-Neto et al., 1993, for evidence that the deafferentation caused disinhibition at the cortical level).

The apparent low-level locus of the plasticity observed by Brasil-Neto et al. is consistent with the mechanisms that are now presumed to underlie the phantom-limb phenomenon (Hall et al., 1990; Cohen et al., 1991a) and provides the most direct evidence to date that the phenomenon is one of central rather than peripheral origin. In a PET experiment, Kew et al. (1994) measured the changes in regional cerebral blood flow correlated with limb movement and TMS-elicited activity in corticospinal neurons in amputees who experienced the phantom-limb phenomenon. Only amputees whose limb removal was due to trauma showed significantly more activity in areas M1 and S1 associated with shoulder movement of the amputated arm compared with the intact arm (figure 7.4) Congenital amputees showed a more normal pattern of activity. The abnormal activity was not limited to the cortex contralateral to the amputation; it also extended to M1 and S1 of the intact arm. TMS in these subjects confirmed the functional relevance of the changes in blood flow. Traumatic but not congenital amputees showed increased corticospinal excitability. These studies show that the reorganization depends on previous experience (increased regional cerebral blood flow and increased excitability in traumatic but not congenital amputees) and that changes occur in different time frames (increased excitability contralateral to amputation in minutes, but not in the ipsilateral cortex).

The phantom-limb phenomenon is often accompanied by a remapping of the amputated limb onto another part of the body. For example, Pascual-Leone et al. (1996) tracked the changes in motor cortex excitability from months before to months after a subject lost his right arm and forearm. In the year following the amputation, the motor output maps of the amputated bicep and of lower facial muscle ipsilateral to the amputated arm expanded over the original representation of the right hand. The expansion was associated with disappearance of phantom sensations and also with the disappearance of the ability of TMS to elicit phantom experience. Figure 7.5 show the progressive changes in the area over which EMG responses can be elicited and the gradual diminution of phantom responses.

The contribution of TMS to the phantom-limb phenomenon is in its infancy, but manipulations of the reorganizing brain of amputees can be used to

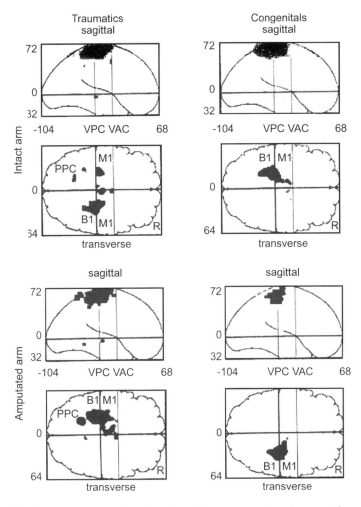

Figure 7.4   Increases in regional cerebral blood flow in traumatic and congenital amputees during shoulder movements of the intact and amputated arm. The traumatic amputees had right-limb amputations, and the congenital amputees had left-arm amputations. In both groups, there was significantly increased blood flow in the motor cortex (M1), the primary so-matosensory cortex (S1), and the supplementary motor cortex contralateral to the amputated arm. The PPC was activated abnormally in the traumatic group but not in the congenital group. The increased blood flow in the traumatic amputees was associated with heightened corticospinal excitability. (From Kew et al., 1994, with permission.)

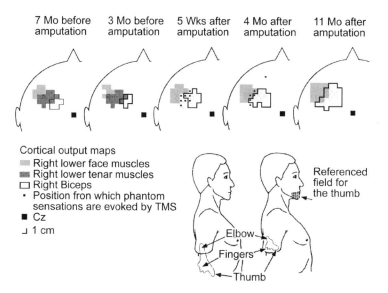

Figure 7.5   Cortical output maps to right-lower face muscles, right thenar muscles, and right biceps obtained by TMS over the motor cortex. The dark spots at five weeks and four months, after traumatic amputation indicate locations where a phantom sensation could be elicited in at least 80% of trials. The lateral views of the body show the drawings of the patient's perception of the phantom at five weeks and four months after the traumatic amputation.

ask many other questions. The reorganization of motor outputs following amputation is not always adaptive, but there are classes of adaptive reorganization that also have been examined with TMS, and it is these classes we examine next.

NECESSITIES FOLLOWING INSUFFICIENCIES

We have made much of the importance of separating brain activity correlated with a behavior from that activity necessary for the behavior, and the same principle applies to assessing the meaning of cortical reorganization. The mere appearance of cortical reorganization does not establish its functional importance.

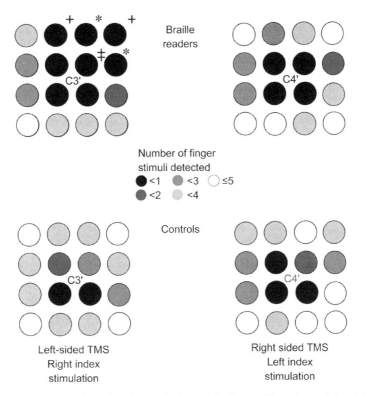

Figure 7.6   Mean number of tactile stimuli detected by five Braille readers and five sighted controls according to scalp position of TMS during the task. (From Pascual-Leone and Torres, 1993, with permission.)

Pascual-Leone and Torres (1993) showed the relationship between the area of cortex devoted to a body representation and the use of the body parts represented. Blind subjects who could read Braille and sighted subjects who could not were given a tactile stimulus–detection task and received TMS over the sites at which somatosensory-evoked potentials had been recorded following electrical stimulation of the index finger. Single-pulse TMS was used and applied at 50 msec after the electrical pulse was delivered to the finger. Figure 7.6 shows the clear difference between the blind and sighted subjects. TMS over the somato-sensory cortex impeded the detection of tactile stimulation over a threefold greater area of the scalp in the blind group. There was also a difference between the dominant and nondominant hands of the Braille readers. TMS over Braille-dominant hands disrupted tactile thresholds over twice as many scalp locations as the nondominant hand of the same subjects. This experiment might allow one to conclude that in the case of blind Braille readers the change in the so-matosensory representation was a consequence of the differential sensory input between the Braille readers' fingers and the sighted subjects', and also between the two hands of the Braille readers. Another possibility is that the effects of so-matosensory TMS were caused by an expansion of the motor cortex due to the repeated finger movements made in reading Braille.

The plasticity observed in the Braille subjects does not mark the end of the reorganization. We emphasized earlier that plasticity is the normal state of the nervous system, so any reorganization due to amputation or blindness would be pointless, if not frankly maladaptive (as in cases of phantom pain), if the new map could not change constantly with the demands of behavior. Evidence of the plasticity of expanded representations of motor areas was seen in a group of blind subjects—all of whom became blind before the age of ten and learned to read Braille before the age of thirteen (Pascual-Leone et al., 1995b). MEPs were recorded from the first dorsal interosseous of both hands and the abductor digiti minimi (ADM, not used for Braille) of the Braille-dominant hand. Figure 7.7 shows the effects of practice with Braille. The subjects read Braille for up to six hours a day at work, but MEP amplitudes diminished markedly after ten days of vacation without much Braille activity. Just one week back at work reinstated the increased amplitude and the number of scalp locations from which a TMS-induced MEP could be elicited. Shorter-term changes in the motor maps also were observed. As figure 7.8 shows, the scalp area from which an MEP could be elicited from the first dorsal interosseous increased in size and sensitivity *during* the working day, but there were no changes on rest days or in the ADM of the Braille-dominant hand.

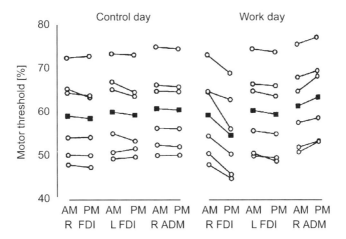

Figure 7.7   Scattergram of motor thresholds for three muscles tested over four testing sessions (morning A.M./afternoon P.M.) on days when subjects were required to use Braille extensively (work day) or to refrain from using Braille (control day). R/L FDI, right/left first dorsal interosseous; R/L ADM, right/left abductor digiti minimi. Threshold is expressed as a percentage of Magstim output. Open circles, individual subjects; filled squares, mean of the six subjects shown. (From Pascual-Leone et al., (1995b) with permission.)

Changes in sensorimotor organization as a result of Braille reading (a sensorimotor activity) are perhaps not too surprising, but there is also evidence that the visual cortex of blind people can be activated by tactile stimuli (Wanet-Defalque et al., 1988; Uhl et al., 1991; Rauscheker, 1995; Pons, 1996; Sadato et al., 1996). The question is whether this activity has a function. We know from physiological studies that visuocortical areas respond to tactile orientation (Haenny, Maunsell and Schiller, 1988; Haenny and Schiller, 1988), but until recently (Zangaladze et al., 1999) it was not clear whether the visual cortex in human subjects could be shown to be necessary for tactile discrimination. We now know that under some circumstances the visual cortex is an aid to tactile perception, and it is possible to view the question of reorganization in blind subjects as one of an unmasking or strengthening previously extant connections and responses. The relevance of the visual cortex for Braille reading was established

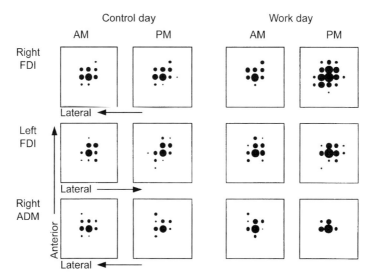

Figure 7.8   Examples of the cortical output maps to the right first dorsal interosseous (FDI) and abductor digiti minimi (ADM) in one subject over four testing sessions on days when Braille was used extensively (work day) for 4–6 hr a day and on nonworking days (control day). The area over which an MEP could be elicited was increased for FDI muscles on work days. (From Pascual-Leone et al., 1995b, with permission.)

by Cohen et al. (1997), who applied TMS to the occipital cortex of blind subjects who were given the task of identifying Braille characters or embossed Roman letters. TMS disrupted tactile performance in the blind subjects but not in sighted controls (figure 7.9). In this study, somatosensory cortex stimulation did not impair tactile discrimination performance in the blind subjects. The explanation offered is that midoccipital TMS causes "interference with more complex discriminative operations performed by occipital cortex in the blind" (1997, 182). This conclusion is at odds, however, both with the earlier demonstration of tactile disruption in blind subjects following somatosensory or motor cortex TMS (Pascual-Leone and Torres, 1993; Pascual-Leone et al., 1995b) and with the suggestion that the occipital activity may explain in part the superior tactile abilities of blind subjects. Indeed, the loss of an essential role for the somatosensory cortex in Braille reading suggested by this study would predict that occipital cortex stimulation should yield a similar change in sensitivity as that observed in the motor cortex (figure 7.9) as a function of short-term practice. It is striking that the visual cortex becomes important for tactile discriminations, but one would expect an emergent interaction or a division of labor between the occipital and somatosensory cortices rather than a loss of the need for somatosensory activity in Braille reading.

TMS is a useful means with which we can approach these questions. Appropriately delivered in time and space, it can disrupt transiently the arrival of the thalamocortical volley of afferent input into the primary sensory cortex and thereby interfere with detection of peripheral somatosensory stimuli (Cohen et al., 1991b). This disruptive effect will result in the subject's failure to detect the stimulus, such that the subject is not aware that he or she received a peripheral somatosensory stimulus prior to TMS. In order to achieve this effect, the magnetic cortical stimulus must be appropriately timed following the peripheral stimulus (Pascual-Leone et al., 1994a). Detection of the peripheral stimulus is disrupted only when the interval between the peripheral stimulus and the cortical stimulus is 15 to 35 msec (Cohen et al., 1991b; Pascual-Leone et al., 1994a). In addition, topographic specificity can be demonstrated according to the known somatotopic organization of the sensory cortex. TMS must be delivered at the appropriate site for projection of index finger afferents when the peripheral stimulus is applied to the index finger pad, and no effect is demonstrable if the site of TMS is displaced by 1 or 2 cm in any direction (Cohen et al., 1991b). These findings provide information about the time course of information arriving to the primary sensory cortex and the processing time in this region in normal subjects.

The same effect of blocking detection of somatosensory stimuli can be demonstrated in blind proficient Braille readers. Pascual-Leone and Torres (1993) reported that detection of electric stimuli applied to the pad of the index finger could be blocked by properly timed TMS to the contralateral sensorimotor cortex. Using a specially designed stimulator that resembled a Braille cell, Pascual-Leone and Torres applied electric stimuli slightly above sensory threshold to the

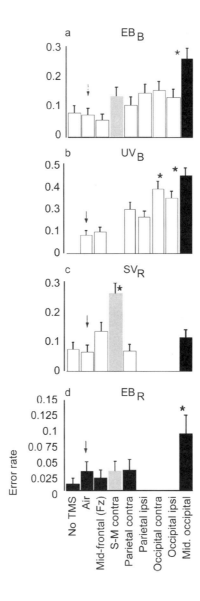

index finger pad of the right or left hand in sighted controls and blind subjects. They followed these peripheral stimuli with TMS stimuli at variable intervals and intensities to different scalp positions targeting the sensorimotor cortex. TMS stimuli appropriately delivered in time and space resulted in a block of detection of the peripheral stimuli such that the subjects were unaware of having received a peripheral stimulus preceding the cortical stimulus.

Pascual-Leone et al. (1998a) used a similar approach to evaluate the timing and contributions of both the somatosensory and occipital cortex to processing of tactile information in blind Braille readers. Real or nonsensical Braille stimuli were presented with a specially designed Braille stimulator to the pad of subjects' reading index fingers. Single-pulse TMS stimuli were applied to the left or right sensorimotor cortex and the striate occipital cortex at variable intervals following the presentation of the Braille stimuli (figure 7.10). TMS presented to the left somatosensory cortex disrupted detection of real and nonsensical Braille stimuli at interstimulus intervals of 20 to 40 msec. At those cortical-peripheral stimulus intervals, the subjects generally did not realize that a peripheral stimulus had been presented. In the instances in which the subjects did realize the

Figure 7.9   Functional relevance of the activation of the occipital cortex for tactile reading in early-blind subjects. The graphs represent error rates (mean + standard error) for the tactile tasks during stimulation of different scalp positions in the four group of subjects studied. Black bars mark the errors induced by stimulation of the midoccipital position, and grey bars the error rates by stimulation of the sensorimotor (S-M)cortex contralateral to the finger used for the tactile task. The different graphs represent the performance of early-blind subjects in Bethesda, Maryland (EB), or in Valencia, Spain (UV), during a task requiring Braille character recognition (subscript B = EB_B, UV_B) or discrimination of embossed Roman letters task (subscript R). Graph c shows the results in a control group of sighted subjects during the embossed Roman-letters task (SV_R). Asterisks mark the positions where significantly more errors occurred than in the baseline condition (discharging TMS off the subjects head = air, marked by arrow). Note that in both tasks blind subjects show significantly greater number of errors during occipital TMS than during any other control condition. In the sighted volunteers, TMS to the occipital cortex had no effect on task performance, whereas the error rate was significantly increased by rTMS to the contralateral sensorimotor cortex. (From Cohen et al., 1997, with permission.)

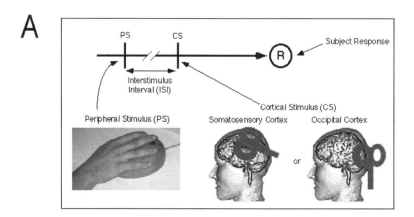

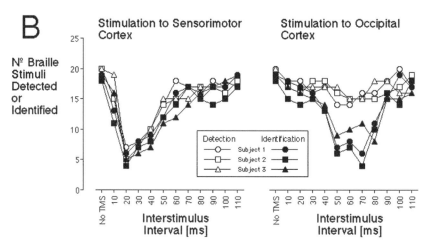

Figure 7.10   Effects of cortical stimulation on specific sites (somatosensory versus striate cortex) during detection and identification of Braille symbols. The figure summarizes the experimental design (*A*) and the results for three early-blind subjects (*B*). The graph displays in open symbols the number of stimuli detected by each subject depending on TMS condition and regardless of whether real or nonsensical Braille stimuli were presented. Filled symbols represent the number of correctly identified Braille stimuli (real versus nonsensical and what Braille character) by each subject depending on TMS condition from among the stimuli that had been detected in the first place. (Adapted from Pascual-Leone et al., 1998a, with permission.)

presentation of a peripheral stimulus, they generally were able to identify correctly whether it was real Braille or not and what Braille symbol was presented. On the other hand, TMS to the striate cortex disrupted the processing of the peripheral stimuli at interstimulus intervals of 50 to 80 msec. Contrary to the findings after sensorimotor TMS, when TMS was applied to the striate cortex, the subjects typically knew whether a peripheral stimulus had been presented or not; therefore, no interference with detection was demonstrated. However, the subjects were unable to discriminate whether the presented stimuli were real or nonsensical Braille or symbols or what particular Braille symbol might have been presented (interference with perception).

Therefore, in early blind subjects, the interval between a tactile stimulus to the finger pad and a cortical stimulus that interferes with processing of tactile information is different for cortical stimulation of the somatosensory and the occipital cortex. This time difference provides insight into the temporal profile of information processing and transfer between somatosensory and striate cortex in early-blind subjects. Two main alternative routes can be entertained: (1) thalamocortical connection to sensory and visual cortex, and (2) cortico-cortical connections from sensory cortex to visual cortex. Although the details of these neural pathways are not yet fully understood, the existing body of data suggests that cortico-cortical connections mediate the cross-modal occipital activity in blind Braille readers. This experiment is a good demonstration of the use of single-pulse TMS for the study of chronometric causality—that is, the inquiry about when in the course of a given task a given brain region becomes critical for behavior.

Plasticity with Practice

The most important type of plasticity we eventually need to understand is not that occurring on a scale of days or hours but on a scale of seconds and milliseconds, the real-time plasticity that allows the brain to meet the changing needs of the external world. We have seen how change occurs in response to injury or abnormality, but it also occurs with something we do every day—repeat familiar acts. Studying how changes occur as a function of practice brings us a little closer to the goal of studying the kind of on-line plasticity discussed earlier in this chapter.

Pascual-Leone, Grafman, and Hallett (1994) showed that changes in motor cortex representation in a learning task were dependent both on the type and stage of learning. Subjects were given a visuomotor response task, and MEPs were measured between blocks of 120 trials (figure 7.11). One group of subjects was given a version of the task in which the location of the stimulus (and thus the finger of response) was randomized from trial to trial, and another group received the trials in a fixed sequence 12 trials long. In the group performing the implicit-sequence learning task, MEP amplitudes increased as subjects became faster in performing the task, and the scalp area over which an MEP could be elicited also increased. When the subjects became fully cognizant of the sequence of finger presses, however, the amplitude and area of the MEPs declined to pretraining levels. Figure 7.12 shows how the two measures were yoked to each other and to the level of performance. The authors concluded that the time course of this modulation of motor cortex activity (a few minutes) was evidence of unmasking of already extant connections between the motor cortex and the more anterior motor-related cortex. Stadler (1994) raised the question of whether this experiment was evidence of a motor involvement in implicit learning or more representative of a strategy of learning. He argued that subjects had foreknowledge of a sequence because they were asked in between trials whether or not they were aware of any sequence. This is likely at least to have engaged explicit search strategies. However, this point does not change the fact that the timing of the motor cortex activity was determined by the subjects' explicit knowledge of the sequence. A more challenging question regarding changes in motor cortex sensitivity surrounds their variability.

In some studies, expansions of cortical maps and increased MEP amplitudes occur simply as a function of a subject making a movement, but other studies have shown practice-specific effects. Classen et al. (1998), for example, measured TMS-evoked responses to stimulation of the cortical representation of the thumb. The direction of the thumb movement elicited by TMS was consistent as shown in

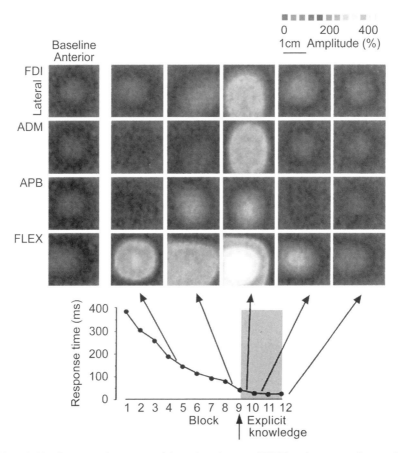

Figure 7.11   Response times on a serial reaction-time test (SRTT) and corresponding cortical output maps for muscles tested in one subject. Complete explicit knowledge of a sequence
of responses was achieved after 9 blocks of 120 trials. The baseline motor output maps were
obtained before the beginning of training. The effects of training on output maps were obtained after blocks 4, 8, 9, 10, and 12 when subjects were at rest. The maps represent contour
plots of the amplitude of the TMS-induced muscle response as a percentage of the maximal
MEP generated over the optimal position at the baseline. (FDI, first dorsal interosseous; ADM,
abductor digiti minimi; APB, abductor policis brevis). Each map encompasses an area 5-by-5
cm centered over the optimal position for activation of each muscle. (From Pascual-Leone et
al., 1994, with permission.)

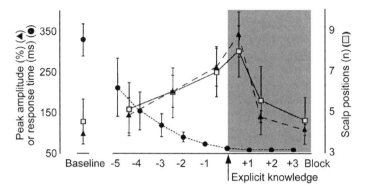

Figure 7.12 Response times on the SRTT task (see Figure 7.11), and peak amplitude and number of scalp positions of the cortical motor output maps for the forearm finger flexors from which TMS-caused MEPs ≥ 60% of the peak amplitude at the baseline. The values express mean ± SD for five test subjects after alignment to the block during which they achieved explicit knowledge. (From Pascual-Leone, Grafman, and Hallett, 1994, with permission.)

figure 7.13. Subjects were then given a simple motor skill–learning task (directed thumb movements in a direction *opposite* to the direction of TMS-evoked thumb movements). TMS was used after training, again to evoke directionally selective thumb movements, but as a result of training cortical stimulation now elicited thumb movements *in the trained direction,* indicating that the organization of thumb representation underwent learning-related changes. To produce this effect, training took place over periods between 5 and 30 min. The direction of thumb movements elicited by TMS after training was monitored to assess the time required for the thumb representation to return to normal. Classen et al. interpreted this result in terms of a short-term memory for movement necessary for the first steps in acquiring motor skills.

Do these studies inform us about some of the changes that might occur outside the motor cortex? The demonstration of the changing role of the parietal cortex in visual search (Walsh, Ashbridge, and Cowey, 1998) is one example of plasticity outside the direct response system. It seems reasonable to suggest that as one makes repeated "target present/absent" responses in search tasks, the

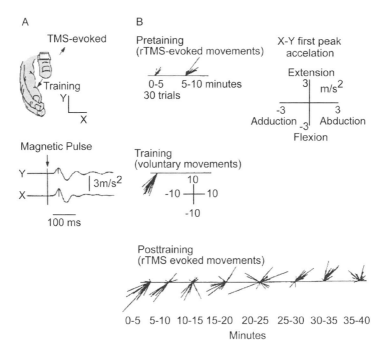

Figure 7.13 The effects of training on cortical representation. TMS was used to evoke thumb movements (*A*) before training. Subjects were then given a training task in which movements were made in the direction opposite to that evoked by TMS. After a few minutes of training, (*B*) TMS applied to the same scalp region as before training elicited thumb movements in the trained rather than the pretrained direction. The bottom trace shows that after training was completed, there was a gradual return to the pretraining response to stimulation of the motor cortex. (From Classen et al., 1998, with permission.)

motor representation of the responding fingers should be affected, and it would be interesting to see if the different cortical areas involved in search change their responses in a set sequence. Take, for example, a visual search task in which the target is a conjunction of movement and form. Performance on this task is disrupted by TMS over V5 (Stewart et al., 1999; Walsh et al., 1999) or over the PPC (Ashbridge, Walsh, and Cowey, 1997; Walsh, Ashbridge, and Cowey, 1998). We also know that the effect of parietal TMS "wears off" as subjects become more efficient at the task. One question is, Does the sensitivity of the motor cortex change in tandem with the loss of the parietal effect? This is tested easily by measuring MEPs at different stages of training. A second question is, Does area V5 change its sensitivity during the same period? Unlike the PPC, the effects of TMS over V5 continue to disrupt filtering of movement despite expertise in the task (Walsh et al., 1999). But this does not preclude changes in V5 activity, and these changes can be measured by taking phosphene thresholds as an analogue of the motor threshold (Stewart et al., 1999; Stewart, Walsh, and Rothwell, 2001). By taking tasks with well-known cortical locations for stimulus and response variables in this way, we can apply to several interacting regions the plasticity that can be measured by TMS.

JUST THE THOUGHT OF IT CHANGES MY BRAIN

Thinking is an act. And if motor acts can change the sensitivity of cortical regions, one might expect thought to have similar effects. If thinking about an event has consequences for the way in which the brain areas involved participate in that event, we again are faced with the seeming impossibility of knowing where in the stream of processing we are making an intervention or taking a measure. We need to know, therefore, how thinking and doing are similar in their effects on the brain and how they differ. Pascual-Leone et al. (1995a) measured changes in motor cortex excitability in subjects who were training on a pianolike exercise. As subjects practiced the keyboard exercise, for 2 hr a day, MEPs from the finger muscles involved could be elicited more easily by TMS. As the subjects practiced over five days, they became faster on the exercise and made fewer errors (figure 7.14). The effects of practice on the motor-output maps can be seen in figure 7.14. The MEPs from the extensor and flexor muscles of the trained hand were obtained from more locations on the scalp contralateral to the hand than could be elicited from the scalp contralateral to the untrained hand. A control group of subjects played the piano at will with their right hand—no sequence information or training instructions were given. The motor maps in this group occupied an intermediate position between the trained hand and the untrained hand of the practice group (figure 7.14). In a

Trained

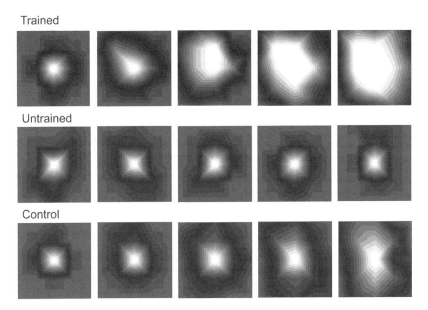

Untrained

Control

Figure 7.14   Examples of cortical motor output maps for the long finger flexor and extensor muscles over five days of training on finger exercises with one hand. Representative cortical maps for a trained, an untrained, and a controlled subject are shown. (From Pascual-Leone et al. 1995a, with permission.)

second experiment, Pascual-Leone et al. asked subjects to practice the piano exercises mentally (without moving their fingers). Structured mental practice produced the same magnitude of change in the motor-output maps as actually practicing the exercises (figure 7.15). The behavioral benefits of the mental rehearsal were almost as great as those of real practice (figure 7.16; see also Mendoza and Wichman, 1978; McBride and Rothstein, 1979).

How far does this phenomenon of mental rehearsal extend to other sensory and cognitive domains? If it is a principle of cortical functioning, then imagining flashes in a certain part of the visual field might be expected to reduce phosphene thresholds in that region, for example. Indeed, Sparing et al. (2002) have recently shown this to be the case. They hypothesized that, analogous to the finding that motor imagery increases the excitability of motor cortex, visual

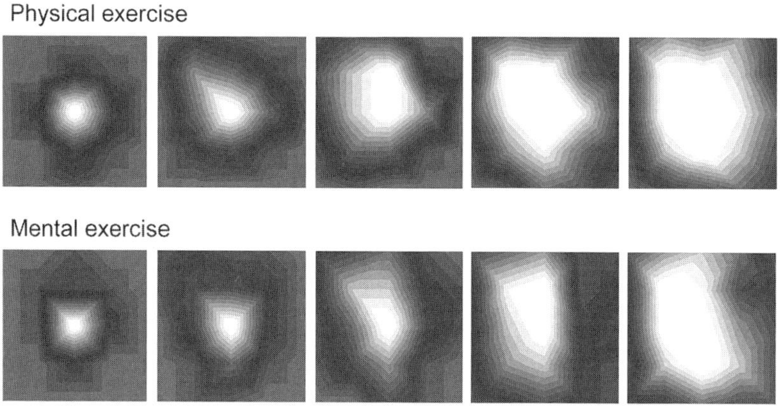

Physical exercise

Mental exercise

Figure 7.15   Examples of cortical motor output maps for the long finger flexor and extensor muscles over five days of physical or mental practice training on the five-finger movement exercise with one hand. (From Pascual-Leone et al., 1995a, with permission.)

imagery should increase visual cortex excitability, as indexed by a decrease in the phosphene threshold. In order to test visual cortex excitability, the primary visual cortex was stimulated with TMS so as to elicit phosphenes in the right-lower visual quadrant. Subjects performed a visual imagery task and an auditory control task. Sparing et al. applied TMS with increasing intensity to determine the phosphene threshold for each subject. Independently of the quadrant in which subjects placed their visual images, imagery decreased phosphene threshold compared to baseline; in contrast, the auditory task did not change phosphene thresholds. These findings demonstrate for the first time a short-term, task-dependent modulation of phosphene thresholds and constitute further evidence that early visual areas participate in visual imagery processing and that mental activity can change cortical brain activity in a measurable way.

There would be limits to the effects of mental practice, of course. Practice is a form of preparation, but being prepared is not all. Bravo and Nakayama (1992) gave an elegant demonstration of how a cognitive or so-called top-down effect could change behavior but not override lower-level perceptual mechanisms. Subjects were presented with a color-discrimination task that required

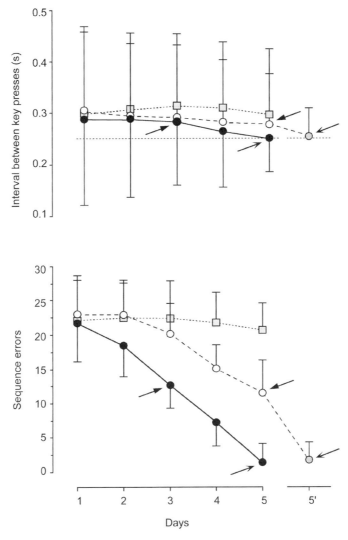

Figure 7.16   Physical and mental practice on a motor learning task have similar effects. The upper graph shows interval between key presses as a function of days of practice. The lower histogram shows the number of errors made on the finger exercise that was either practiced or imagined. Filled circles, physical practice group; open circles, mental practice group; squares, control group; circle at 5′, mental practice group on day five. (From Pascual-Leone et al., 1995a, with permission.)

them to detect the presence of a particular red or green target. The target could be either red or green on any trial, and if the color target was the same as on a previous trial, the reaction time was faster than if the color target was different from the previous trial—in other words, a stimulus-specific priming effect. If subjects were informed of the simple sequence of stimulus targets—say, two reds followed by two greens, two reds, two greens, and so on—such that the subjects knew exactly which target was going to appear on the next trial, they were, of course, faster overall on the task. But the foreknowledge of the target, although affecting baseline reaction time, had no effect on the priming; subjects were still faster on the second red and second green of each pair than on the first of each pair. It would be interesting to see if mental practice of this task would produce the same effects as foreknowledge of the stimuli—that is, a baseline change but no effect on the dynamics of priming. TMS over the appropriate visual area under conditions in which the subject knows which target is coming next would also be a way of assessing the level at which the critical information was stored (see Bisley and Pasternak, 2000; Campana, Cowey, and Walsh, 2002). How an analogue of this experiment would work in the motor system would also be an interesting test of the power of mental practice observed in Pascual-Leone et al.'s study of piano exercises. Do the specific effects on performance in that study suggest more than a raise in baseline activity? It would seem more parsimonious to suggest that neither mental nor real practice can override the moment-to-moment dynamics of behavior; indeed, there should be a cost when the task diverges from that practiced. These and similar experiments show how TMS can be used to combine medium-term changes in brain activity (e.g., motor maps) with short-term demands for changes in performance to examine the dynamic interactions between different levels of information processing, including expectation and rehearsal.

GUIDING CHANGE

TMS is not limited to measuring change; it also can induce cortical plasticity and in doing so offer the possibility of therapeutic applications. One recent study has demonstrated that TMS applied to motor regions can be used to affect the degree of learning in an implicit motor-learning task (Pascual-Leone et al., 1999b). Specifically, Pascual-Leone and colleagues found that 1 Hz stimulation had a deleterious effect on learning, whereas 10 Hz stimulation had a positive effect (Tarazona et al., 1997; Pascual-Leone, Grafman, and Hallett, 1994). The task used in this study was the same as that used by Pascual-Leone, Grafman, and Hallett, in their 1994 study of implicit learning, but in the 1999 experiment TMS was applied before the blocks of learning. As figure 7.17 shows, 1 Hz stimulation over the motor cortex impeded the implicit learning of the sequence, whereas 10 Hz rTMS over the dorsolateral prefrontal cortex enhanced learning. There is good agreement that 1 Hz stimulation reduces activity in cortex but less agreement that 10 Hz increases activity (see chapter 3). In terms of the neural noise concept, the 1 Hz stimulation over the motor cortex can be said to have disrupted the changes in motor areas observed in the earlier study (Pascual-Leone, Grafman, and Hallett, 1994). The enhancing effect of 10 Hz over the dorsolateral prefrontal cortex is more difficult to explain, but one possibility is that dorsolateral prefrontal cortex learning involves a consolidation period in the intertrial intervals, during which time the 10 Hz stimulation may have operated in a long-term potentiation–like manner, whereas the association underlying learning in the motor cortex occurs only during the execution of the task when the stimulation was active and therefore disruptive.

Stewart et al. (1999) carried out a similar experiment, showing how TMS can affect learning in the visual system. Moving phosphenes were evoked by stimulation of an area of the scalp overlying the likely location of visual area V5. This extrastriate moving phosphene area was then used as the site for TMS given to two groups of subjects during learning of a motion-detection task. The two groups received either 3 Hz or 10 Hz stimulation on every trial of the task as they carried it out. The rTMS began at the onset of the visual array and continued for one second. The intensity used was 80% of phosphene threshold (range between 35% [0.7 Tesla] and 56% [1.12 Tesla] of stimulator output), a level that would be likely to stimulate V5 without overtly disrupting function (and that did not elevate reaction times). The rationale for using 80% was adapted from motor

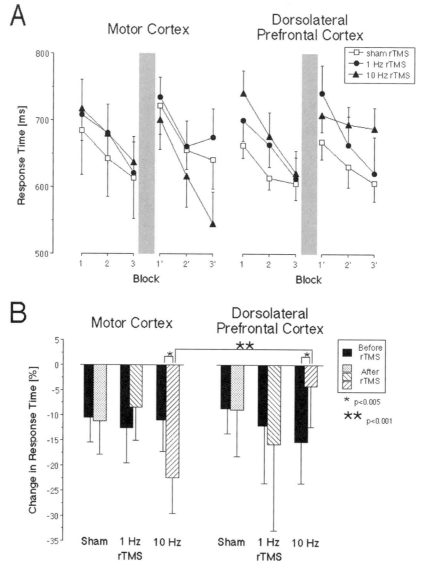

Figure 7.17 Effects of modulation of excitability of motor or contralateral dorsolateral prefrontal cortex by rTMS on procedural learning in a serial reaction-time task. The top graph (*A*) shows average response times for all subjects during three blocks of learning before and after delivery of rTMS (1 Hz or 10 Hz or sham). Visual stimuli were presented in a repeating sequence, of which the subjects were unaware. The lower graph (*B*) shows the change in response time from block 1 to 3 as an index of implicit procedural learning. Data are means ± Standard deviation. (From Pascual-Leone et al., 1999b, with permission.)

studies in which the motor threshold is used as a guide for the level of stimulation to be applied (e.g., Rothwell, 1993; Berardelli et al., 1994; Kew et al., 1994; Lemon, Johansson, and Westling, 1995; Pascual-Leone et al., 1999). Figure 7.18 shows that the group receiving 3 Hz learned significantly less than both a control group and the 10 Hz group, which did not differ from each other. The two important aspects of this result are a correspondence between the effects of low-frequency stimulation over both the motor cortex and the visual cortex and the dissociation of TMS effects on a single trial from cumulative effects over many trials.

Stefan et al. (2000) measured TMS-evoked MEP amplitudes from the right abductor pollicis brevis and then paired a low-frequency, suprathreshold electrical stimulus to the right median nerve with a single pulse (120% of motor threshold) over the left motor cortex. This paired stimulus was repeated ninety times with various median nerve-TMS onset asynchronies. When MEPs to a fixed TMS value were measured after this intervention, the amplitude increase was significant compared with prestimulation levels. They successfully showed an association between sensory and magnetic stimuli. Stefan et al. argued on several grounds that the site of this associative change in motor excitability was cortical: F-waves elicited by stimulation of the median nerve remained unaffected by the intervention (see also Ugawa et al., 1991); and the silent period, assumed to be at least in part cortically generated (Hallett, 1995), was lengthened by the intervention. The induced plasticity evolved rapidly, was persistent but reversible, relied on the precise temporal relationship of the stimulus pairing, and was topographically specific—all features consistent with long-term potentiation–like mechanisms.

IS THE CHAOS IMPENETRABLE?

What we have seen in this chapter is the ability of TMS to probe the dynamics of change from a time span of years to a time window of milliseconds. We also have seen that the mechanisms of plasticity can be probed by using TMS as a primary lesion, as a secondary lesion, or as a stimulant to modulate plasticity. With

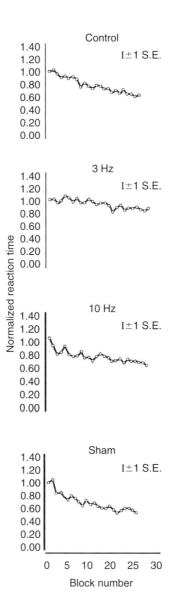

two exceptions (Walsh et al., 1998a, 1999), all the studies of plasticity discussed in this chapter have been studies of changes in the input of the somatosensory or visual cortices or in the output of the motor cortex. For cognitive neuropsychology, these studies can constitute only the hint of a beginning of interesting work in plasticity. In terms of the need to understand on-line plasticity, some beginnings can be seen in studies of priming (Campana, Cowey, and Walsh, 2002), expectation (Ellison, Rushworth, and Walsh, submitted), and the effects of very short-term practice (Classen et al., 1998). We are faced here with the same problem Penfield and his coworkers faced when stimulating the brain electrically (Penfield and Rasmussen, 1950). It was relatively easy to elicit movements, sounds, or sights, but what Penfield termed the "elaboration areas" didn't have such salient and easily reproducible signatures of activity. Those researchers studying cognitive plasticity now need to find ways of exploring these elaboration areas and their role in and modulation by on-line plasticity. One intriguing possibility, of course, is that on-line plasticity is neither under the control of any single area nor under top-down control, but is simply a feature of short-term changes in the activity of sensory and motor neurons. For example, Maljkovic and Nakayama (1994) have provided a convincing account of visual priming in terms of a number of separate independent mechanisms responding to color, movement, contour space, and so on, and their account might extend to other domains.

Figure 7.18   Effects of two frequencies of rTMS on learning a visual motion-discrimination task in a search paradigm. Repetitive TMS was delivered during the training period at either 3 Hz or 10 Hz as subjects performed the motion search task. The data are normalized to the reaction times on Block 1 (first baseline without TMS), and further baselines without TMS were taken after 12 blocks of 50 trials, over three days, with TMS delivered on every trial and again after a further 8 blocks of 50 over days three and four. The baselines are indicated by open symbols. The control group (*top*) who did not receive TMS improved reaction times by almost 0.4 of the first baseline, as did the 10 Hz group and the sham-treated group. TMS at 3 Hz, however, delayed the learning significantly. S.E., Standard error. (From Stewart et al., 1999, with permission.)

CAN I BORROW YOUR ILLNESS?

In April 1861, a fifty-one-year-old man was admitted to the surgical service at the Bicetre hospital in Paris with an extensive infection of his right leg (McHenry, 1969). The physician in charge, Pierre Paul Broca (1824–80; figure 8.1) was a surgeon and an anthropologist who had studied Cro-Magnon man and neolithic trephination and who eventually established the world's first Anthropological Society and his own School and Institute of Anthropology. Broca amputated the patient's leg, but despite his efforts the man died a week later. Broca performed an autopsy, including an examination of the patient's brain, and the next day demonstrated before the Anthropological Society the brain lesion of this patient with a nonfluent speech disorder that he named *aphémie* (from *a* = not and *phéme* = voice). The patient, nicknamed "Tan," had lost his ability to speak at age thirty. He was able to understand and communicate by gestures but could utter only the monosyllabic expression "tan, tan, tan"—hence, his nickname. Tan was able to work and care for himself, but in his forties he developed weakness of his right arm and later of his right leg and became bedridden. Broca knew of Jean Baptiste Bouillaud, professor of clinical medicine at the Charité in Paris, who in 1827 had offered 500 francs to whoever might demonstrate that speech disorders were associated with lesions other than in the left frontal lobe of the brain. In the 1820s, Bouillaud made extensive

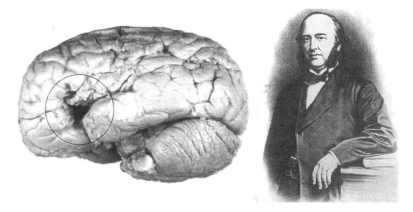

Figure 8.1   Pierre Paul Broca demonstrating the lesion in the left frontal operculum of Tan's brain.

clinical and pathological studies and concluded: "It is necessary to distinguish two different phenomena in the act of speech, namely, the power of creating words as signs of our ideas and that of articulating these same words." Bouillaud was sure that the latter phenomenon was localized to the left frontal lobe—hence, his money offer. Broca had called upon Ernest Auburtin, Bouillaud's son-in-law, to examine patient Tan and to consult with him about the localization of the brain lesion that might have led to Tan's speech problem and right-side weakness. Eventually, when Tan developed the infection of the right leg that brought him to Broca's care and that led to his death, Broca must have seen the opportunity to resolve a burning question in anthropology and neurology regarding the brain correlates of speech. This constitutes one of the first and best-known examples of borrowing a patient's illness to address a fundamental question in cognitive neuroscience. Tan's leg infection is now generally unknown, whereas his speech disorder and associated brain lesion are widely recognized. In the 1870s, Sir David Ferrier, the Scottish neurophysiologist and chairman of neuropathology at King's College in London who pioneered the concept of localization of function in the brain, eventually named the third left

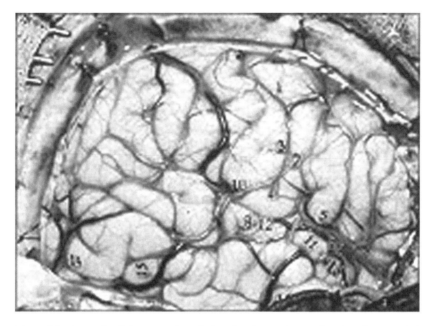

Figure 8.2   Example of the exposed cortical surface in a patient undergoing direct cortical mapping during the evaluation for epilepsy surgery. The numbers mark sites identified to be associated with various motor, sensory, and cognitive functions. See Penfield and Jasper, 1954, for details.

frontal convolution *Broca's area,* and so the "softening" of the third frontal convolution of Tan's left brain hemisphere has become a classic piece of evidence of brain localization and neural organization of language (figure 8.1).

Borrowing a patient's illness has become a standard mode of operation to address cognitive neuroscience questions. Cortical stimulation studies in epileptic patients undergoing presurgical evaluation, as popularized by Wilder Penfield (figure 8.2) at the Montreal Neurological Institute (Penfield and Jasper, 1954), illustrate this approach particularly well. Patients with medication-resistant epilepsy can be helped by resection of the epileptogenic tissue. However, this procedure requires precise localization of the seizure focus and careful

assessment of the function of the surrounding brain tissue to rule out the possibility that surgical resection might lead to serious cognitive, sensory, or motor
deficits. Brain mapping and direct cortical stimulation techniques are used for
this purpose. The patient's brain is exposed, and with the patient awake, cortical
sites are electrically stimulated and the induced phenomena noted (figure 8.2).
Alternatively, subdural electrode arrays are implanted, and during the following
few days the patients are monitored carefully, and the effects of stimulation by
the different subdural electrodes are assessed (Lesser et al., 1987). In any case,
these interventions, required for proper surgical planning, provide a unique opportunity to study a variety of cognitive functions, and over the past fifty years
much has been learned about brain-behavior correlations thanks to the opportunities for borrowing the illness of epileptic patients and for studying cognitive
phenomena beyond those strictly required for clinical care.

Lesion studies are another example of how we piggyback on a patient's illness to investigate brain-behavior relations. Milner's studies on patient H.M.,
who following resection of the temporal lobes became amnestic, not only served
the purpose of helping the patient, his family, and physicians understand the
clinical deficit that H.M. presented, but also shaped the field of cognitive neuroscience of memory (Milner, 1966; Milner, Squire, and Kandel, 1998). The dissociation of memory systems for declarative and procedural memory and their
representation in separate processing streams in the brain followed Milner's careful dissection of H.M.'s deficits. The railway construction foreman Phineas Gage
provided critical clues about the contributions of frontal areas to behavior. Gage
was twenty-five years old when in a bizarre accident the tamping iron he was
using to trigger controlled explosions to level uneven terrain for the laying
of new rail tracks was hurled, projectile-like, through his face, skull, and brain
(figure 8.3). Gage survived but underwent dramatic changes in his personality
that captured the interest of his physician, John Harlow. Twenty years after the
accident, Harlow carefully reported his patient's behavioral change, correlating
them with the presumed area of damage in the brain (Harlow, 1868). Gage died
in 1861, and no autopsy was performed, but his skull and the tamping iron that
caused his brain injury were recovered (figure 8.3). Almost a century after

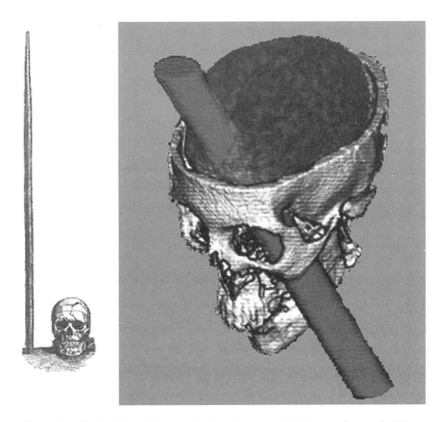

Figure 8.3   Gage's skull and the tamping iron that caused his injury, as kept at the Warren Anatomical Museum in Boston. His reconstructed skull and brain demonstrate the regions damaged by the rod. (Modified from Damasio et al., 1994.)

Gage's death, with the benefit of the body of knowledge in neuropsychology and cognitive neuroscience that Harlow did not have, Damasio and colleagues (1994) reconstructed Gage's brain from measurements of his skull and the tamping iron (figure 8.3), shedding light on the role of prefrontal cortical areas in rational decision making and emotional processing.

Such landmark patients demonstrate how the careful study of their problems beyond the strict requirements of their examination for the purposes of

clinical care and treatment can aid in advancing our knowledge of brain function and provide unique opportunities to test theories and concepts. TMS
studies in patients can enhance our understanding about the pathophysiology
of their disease, help establish a prognosis of the clinical course, and possibly
guide pharmacologic interventions (Hallett, 1996). For example, studies of corticospinal responses to motor cortex TMS in patients with a hemiparesis following a stroke suggest that measurements of amplitude and latency of the
MEPs might be useful in assessing clinical prognosis and in illuminating the
different mechanisms of motor recovery (preservation of projections, unmasking of latent connections, shifts in intracortical excitability, or recruitment of
alternative pathways) (Catano et al., 1996; Catano, Houa, and Noel, 1997;
Rossini and Rossi, 1998; Muellbacher, Artner, and Mamoli, 1999; Caramia
et al., 2000; Trompetto et al., 2000). Studies of motor cortical excitability in some
patients with medication-refractory major depression reveal interhemispheric
asymmetries in motor threshold and paired-pulse curves with reduced excitability in the left hemisphere, which may be predictive of clinical response
to treatment (Maeda et al., 2000; Maeda and Pascual-Leone, in press). In patients with congenital mirror movements, mapping of the motor output with
TMS demonstrates the presence of ipsilateral hand responses to motor cortex
stimulation, proving that aberrant organization of motor representation areas
and corticospinal pathways with ipsilateral as well as contralateral control of
voluntary movements underlies the behavioral disorder (Konogaya, Mano, and
Konogaya, 1990; Cohen et al., 1991). In patients with migraine, TMS to the
occipital cortex can be used to evoke phosphenes and to confirm the hyperexcitability of the visual cortex in the migraine interictum, both in patients
with and without aura (van der Kamp et al., 1996; Afra et al., 1998; Aurora
et al., 1998; Mulleners et al., 2001). In patients with focal dystonia, studies
of cortico-cortical excitability demonstrate a reduced intracortical inhibition
(Ridding et al., 1995; Chen et al., 1997), thus providing critical clues about the
pathophysiology of the abnormal control of motor tone. Finally, in patients
with epilepsy, abnormalities of intracortical excitability can be documented
that may account for the risk of epileptic discharges and seizure generalization

and thus may guide the choice of the antiepileptic medication best suited for a given patient based on the effects different agents have on cortical excitability (Ziemann et al., 1998). The list of diseases in which similar studies have been conducted is long, and it is not our aim to be exhaustive. Further details on these potential clinical uses of TMS can be found elsewhere (Mills, 1999; Pascual-Leone et al., 2001).

We have argued that TMS virtual lesions allow one to address brain-behavior relations without the constraints of other lesion or cortical stimulation techniques (see chapters 1, 4, and 5). Lesion studies depend on the caprice by which one may come across a patient in whom one might be able to test a concept, such as Broca with patient Tan. For this reason, lesion studies often are limited to a single case: the lesion might be larger than the brain region of interest; there might be more than a single lesion; or the lesion might have caused more global cognitive deficits, making it difficult to test the patient carefully. The patient's lesion frequently will have occurred long before the time of study, such that reorganization of brain functions and plasticity may have changed the cortical organization and the brain-behavior relationship under study (Robertson and Murre, 1999). Cortical stimulation studies are equally problematic because patients have abnormal brain substrates; there are time constraints on the tests, which are conducted in the rather stressful surroundings of an operating room; and the patient is necessarily worried and anxious given the impending brain surgery. Using TMS puts one in a position to create patients rather than to borrow a patient's illness, but these two approaches can be combined by taking TMS to patients and illustrating the additional insights that can be gained by doing so.

COMPENSATORY ANALYSIS

In previous chapters, we discussed the logic and limits of lesion analysis and the role TMS has in combining spatial and temporal factors in virtual lesions. In 1989, Hanna Damasio and Antonio Damasio defended the lesion analysis method and offered a useful adaptation of it for neuroimaging. In their words,

"The essence of the lesion method is the establishment of a correlation between a circumscribed region of damaged brain and changes in some aspect of an experimentally controlled behavioral performance" (1989). More important, as they pointed out, "the distinction between the possible and accurate localization of damage . . . and the nonlocalizability of complex psychological functions [are] critical." Lomber (1999), whose own work relies on reversible lesions induced by cooling the cortex, pointed out that if one removes a brain area experimentally or examines a patient who has suffered permanent brain damage, then one is studying the function of the tissue that remains. The injury can be localized anatomically, and the behavior can be measured precisely, but the latter is the consequence of the workings of the residual brain. That is not to say that the remaining tissue or the behavior is normal. Damage to a brain area also incurs damage to distal sites by severing vessels, ablating white matter, and degenerating neurons along the tracts serving the removed area. Similarly, temporary disruption of cortical brain function by TMS not only affects the directly targeted brain region, but also exerts distant, trans-synaptic effects. As discussed in chapters 4 and 9, the combination of TMS with neuroimaging or EEG provides a method of demonstrating such remote effects. However, the role that such distant effects of TMS might have on the behavior being assessed remains to be ascertained. The primate brain seems to be a mosaic of highly interconnected, spatially distributed, and distinct regions. Lesions of these cortico-cortical and cortico-subcortical connections result in specific neurological and psychiatric "dysconnection" syndromes. Therefore, human brain function and behavior seem best explained on the basis of functional connectivity between brain structures rather than on the basis of localization of a given function to a specific brain structure. This approach to explaining normal behavior and neuropsychiatric disorders at the level of distributed neural networks requires a technique for identification of how cortico-cortical and cortico-subcortical connectivity changes in vivo while the subject performs a task. In addition, as argued in earlier chapters, the causal role of such changes with a given behavior can be established only by an intervention that disrupts activity in critical nodes of the network.

Mottaghy et al. (2000) studied the effects of rTMS of the prefrontal cortex as subjects performed a 2-back working-memory task. TMS to the right or left dorsolateral prefrontal cortex, but not to the midline frontal cortex, significantly worsened performance in the task, hence establishing the causal role of these regions for the behavior under study. Disruption of task performance was measured as a change in reaction time, and TMS to the left and right dorsolateral prefrontal cortex lengthened reaction time by a similar amount. Therefore, it would appear that both of these areas contribute similarly to the 2-back task studied. However, Mottaghy et al. conducted the study while measuring changes in regional cerebral blood flow as revealed by PET (figure 8.4). The changes in task performance following TMS to the right and the left dorsolateral prefrontal cortex were associated with similar reduction in the regional cerebral blood flow in the targeted brain regions but had different effects on distant brain areas. Residual task performance during the TMS-induced disruption of the right and left dorsolateral prefrontal cortex is related to the capacity of the brain to react to the temporary lesion, and differential effects of left and right prefrontal TMS must account for the differences in brain activity in that setting. Task performance during TMS to the left dorsolateral prefrontal cortex was associated, as compared with baseline performance during sham stimulation, with decreased regional cerebral blood flow in that targeted area. On the other hand, task performance during TMS to the right dorsolateral prefrontal cortex was associated with decreased regional cerebral blood flow in that targeted area, but also in the left dorsolateral prefrontal cortex and the bilateral parietal cortices (figure 8.4). A correlation analysis of the change in cerebral blood flow and of the behavioral disruption as indexed by the change in reaction time shows that whether TMS is applied to the right or the left dorsolateral prefrontal cortex, the change in left-sided activity is the most critical predictor of the behavioral effects.

ADDING INSULT TO INJURY

An alternative way to study brain-behavior relations at the level of compensatory analysis is to take TMS to patients with focal brain lesions and assess how the

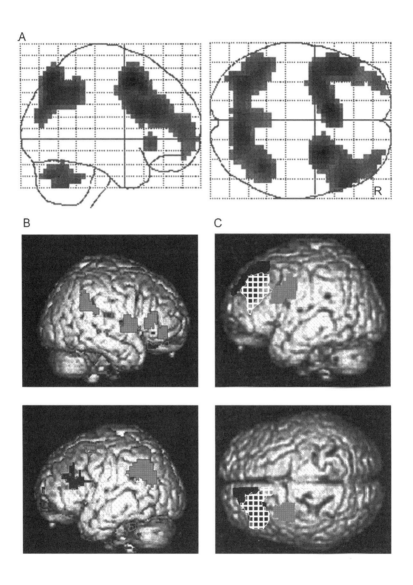

lesion changes the effects of TMS of a specific cortical target on performance in a given task, as compared with TMS in subjects without such lesions or in patients with lesions in other sites. The unpredictability of nature sometimes allows a similar level of analysis. For example, some patients recover from the aphasia that can follow a stroke, and the mechanisms of such recovery are a matter of debate. Functional imaging studies suggest activation of compensatory areas, including a role of right hemispheric structures, but they cannot establish a causal relation between activity in the nondominant hemisphere and language function. It is conceivable that the brain lesion of the dominant hemisphere that caused the aphasia also might lead to a disinhibition of distant brain regions that may show activation on functional imaging studies representing an epiphenomenon, rather than being causally related to the recovery of speech. Bartolomeo et al. (1998) reported a seventy-four-year-old woman who had partially recovered reading ability, becoming a letter-by-letter reader following a left hemispheric

---

Figure 8.4   Spatial distribution of regional cerebral blood-flow changes while subjects perform a 2-back working memory task with or without concurrent TMS to the right or left dorsolateral prefrontal cortex. In (*A*), the spatial distributions of significantly activated voxels are shown as integrated projections along sagittal and axial axes while subjects performed the working memory task during sham TMS (R, right). The voxels show levels of significance above a threshold of $p = 0.001$ and a cluster size of $k = 20$ (SPM glass brain projections). In (*B*), the deactivations induced by rTMS of the left (green) and the right (blue) dorsolateral prefrontal cortex are shown as an overlay on a 3-D surface–rendered anatomical magnetic resonance image ($p < 0.01; k = 20$). Note that deactivations induced by left-sided rTMS (green) are limited to the frontal region directly targeted by TMS. However, deactivation during rTMS to the right hemisphere presents at the prefrontal site of stimulation, the bilateral parietal cortices, and the left dorsolateral prefrontal region. Despite these differences in cerebral blood-flow results, the behavioral effects of right and left prefrontal rTMS, as indexed by the changes in response time, were not statistically different. (*C*) shows the overlay of the negative correlations between regional cerebral blood flow and performance (as indexed by the response time) in the 2-back working memory task. Red represents the trials without rTMS; green, those during rTMS to the left dorsolateral prefrontal cortex; and blue, those during rTMS to the right prefrontal cortex. Regardless of the site of rTMS (right or left), the disruption of left-sided prefrontal activity is the only one correlated with task performance. (Modified from Mottaghy et al., 2000.)

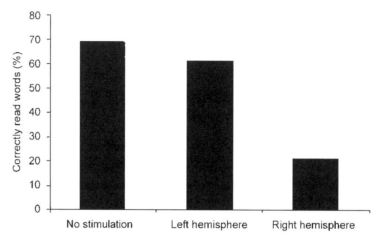

Figure 8.5 Effect of TMS on oral reading during left or right hemispheric stimulation expressed as number of words read correctly. Note the dramatic effect of right hemispheric TMS: a marked decrease in performance. (Modified from Coslett and Monsul, 1994, with permission.)

hematoma. A second, mirror-image hematoma in the right hemisphere seven months later led to significant worsening of her reading ability both in terms of accuracy and reading latency for words and isolated letters. TMS might be used favorably to explore such patterns of effects. In 1994, using TMS, Coslett and Monsul tested the hypothesis that the right hemisphere mediates the preserved reading ability in some patients with acquired dyslexia by transiently disrupting right hemispheric structures. Essentially, their study represents a predictor of what nature eventually allowed Bartolomeo et al. to study in their 1998 patient. Coslett and Monsul asked their patient with partially recovered pure alexia to read aloud some words briefly presented, half of which were shown in association with TMS of the right or left hemisphere (figure 8.5). Consistent with the right-hemisphere reading hypothesis, stimulation of the right but not the left hemisphere disrupted oral reading. One might envision a systematic follow-up study to such pioneering work. Functional MRI of patients with recovered or partially recovered language abilities following strokes of the dominant hemisphere would provide information about the right-hemisphere areas to target with TMS, which might then be used to disrupt function of those brain regions transiently and evaluate their role in the recovery of language.

A series of studies on spatial attention and neglect provide further examples of this approach. Oliveri et al. (1999) elegantly illustrate the potential of TMS in providing chronometric information of the causal role of a given cortical region for a behavior (chapter 6). They used TMS in a tactile stimulus–detection task to demonstrate that the right, but not the left, parietal cortex is critical for detection not only of contralateral but also of ipsilateral stimuli. They found that bimanual discrimination is disrupted more readily than unimanual tasks, but only by right parietal TMS. Most important, they showed that the contribution of the right parietal cortex takes place approximately 40 msec after the tactile stimuli are applied, hence suggesting involvement of late cortical events. Fierro et al. (2000) extended these results, showing that TMS not only can induce extinction to simultaneous visual stimulation of the two hemifields, but also can correct pseudoneglect. The neurophysiology of extinction might in fact be different than that of neglect, the latter being of greater clinical significance (Kinsbourne, 1994; Bisiach et al., 1996; Vallar, 1998). Patients with neglect face tremendous difficulties in rehabilitation because they do not realize the extent of their own limitations. We hope that understanding neglect better will aid in developing suitable methods for its treatment. Oliveri's and Fierro's results seem to support the widespread notion that the right hemisphere contains representations of both hemispaces, whereas the left hemisphere is concerned with attending only to the contralateral hemispace. However, interhemispheric competition (possibly asymmetrical) of cortical or subcortical structures might be better suited to explain some of these effects. Only interhemispheric competition provides a plausible explanation for the puzzling effects, extensively studied in cats, by which visual hemineglect induced by a lesion of one posterior cortex paradoxically can be reversed by secondary damage to contralateral cortical and subcortical structures (Lomber and Payne, 1996). Using exactly the same logic, Oliveri et al. (1999) have used TMS to test this notion in twenty-eight patients with right ($n = 14$) or left ($n = 14$) brain lesions. Single-pulse TMS was delivered to frontal and parietal scalp sites of the unaffected hemisphere 40 msec after application of a unimanual or bimanual electric-digit stimulus. In patients with right hemispheric damage, left frontal TMS significantly reduced the rate of contralateral extinctions compared with controls. Left parietal TMS did not affect the number of extinctions significantly as compared with baseline. Left-brain-damaged patients did not show equivalent results. In them, TMS to the intact, right hemisphere did not alter the recognition of bimanual stimuli. TMS to the left frontal cortex in patients with right hemispheric lesions significantly reduced the rate of contralateral extinctions, even though, as mentioned earlier, the same type of stimulation did not affect task performance in normal subjects. These results suggest that extinctions produced by right-hemisphere damage may be dependent on a breakdown in the balance of hemispheric rivalry in directing spatial attention to the contralateral hemispace, so that the unaffected hemisphere generates an unopposed orienting response to the side with the lesion (figure 8.6). TMS to the left frontal cortex in patients with right-hemisphere damage and contralesional extinction ameliorates their deficit. The mechanism of action of TMS in this setting might involve crossed frontoparietal inhibition. However, interactions at the subcortical level cannot be excluded.

Evaluation of cortico-cortical pathways can be conducted using paired-pulse stimulation (Kujirai et al., 1993; Ziemann, Rothwell, and Ridding, 1996). Following their study of right-brain-damaged patients with neglect, Oliveri et al. (2000) used paired-pulse TMS to induce selective intracortical inhibition or facilitation of the unaffected hemisphere depending on the interstimulus interval. The hypothesis was that cortical inhibition would result in improvement and cortical facilitation in a worsening of contralesional extinction as compared with baseline. Paired-pulse TMS with the interstimulus interval set at 1 msec or 10 msec was applied to the left parietal or frontal cortex at various intervals following bimanual electric-digit stimulation. At an interstimulus interval of 1 msec, which leads to intracortical inhibition, paired-pulse TMS led to a greater improvement in extinction than that induced by single-pulse TMS

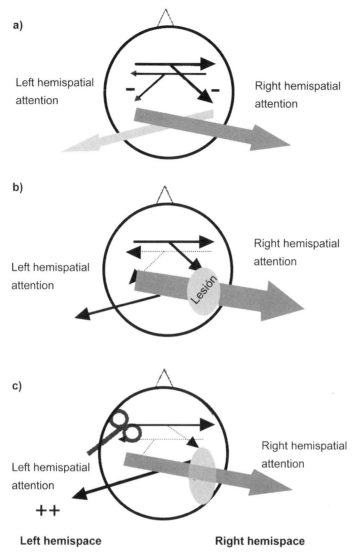

Left hemispace   **Right hemispace**

Figure 8.6   Proposed framework for left and right hemispheric contributions to the neural representation of egocentric space. In normal volunteers (*a*), the mutual inhibitory callosal connections between the two hemispheres are asymmetric, with the dominant hemisphere exerting greater inhibition onto the nondominant hemisphere, hence producing a slight hyperorientation to the right side. Following a right-hemisphere stroke (*b*), the unbalanced effect of the left hemisphere results in excessive attention toward the right (ipsilesional) hemispace (dashed arrow). In right brain–damaged patients (*c*), left frontal TMS interferes with the hypothesized left frontal/right parietal inhibition, thus disinhibiting the right parietal cortex and partially restoring left extinctions (black arrow). (Modified from Oliveri et al., 1999b.)

(Oliveri et al., 1999) (figure 8.7). On the other hand, with paired-pulse TMS at 10 msec, which is believed to increase cortical facilitation, there was a worsening of extinction as compared with baseline, completely reversing the effects of single-pulse TMS (figure 8.7). These results shed further light on the mechanisms of tactile extinction. In addition, this study illustrates the potential of paired-pulse TMS to modulate intracortical excitability selectively and to extend the results of single-pulse TMS.

Such studies provide evidence of the dynamic changes and adaptation that take place in the human brain following a brain injury; they thus connect with the line of evidence regarding plasticity of the brain that we discussed in chapter 7. Lesions do not have to affect the central nervous system. For example, four-week immobilization of hand and arm following traumatic wrist fractures results in changes in cortical output maps with increases in cortical excitability presumably due to the combined effects of restriction in volitional movements and changes in the somatosensory and proprioceptive inputs (Zanette et al., 1997). In addition, such studies allow one to address behavior at the level of compensatory analysis and paradoxical lesion effects (Kapur, 1996). In the case of neglect, the possibility of resolving deficits by applying TMS to the healthy hemisphere would be of profound importance in the neurorehabilitation of patients with right parietal lesions, and in general such findings alert us to the potential therapeutic effects of TMS.

Application of TMS serially to different cortical areas may allow one to model such effects. For example, 1 Hz rTMS to the right parietal lobe results in contralateral neglect for a period of several minutes following stimulation (Hilgetag et al., 2001). During this time, ipsilateral attention is enhanced by the imbalance in interhemispheric competition created by the transient virtual lesions induced by TMS (Hilgetag et al., 2001). Furthermore, it should be possible, in this period of time following the rTMS, to apply a second train of TMS to the left hemisphere and to assess the effects of bihemispheric modulation, hence using the first rTMS application as a model of patients with a right hemispheric lesion and the second TMS as a probe of the compensatory modulation of brain function. A similar approach can be taken to model patients with cerebellar

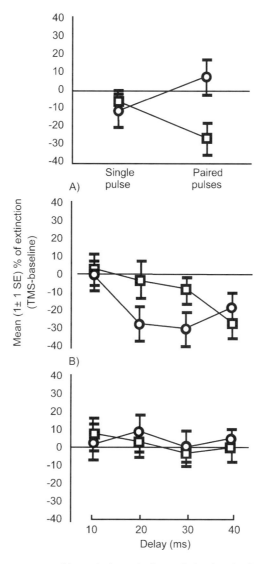

Figure 8.7   Mean percentage (± standard error) of contralesional extinction for single-pulse and paired-pulse TMS paradigms. Results express the difference between baseline and TMS conditions. Trials with paired-pulse TMS at 1 msec (squares) and 10 msec (circles) show divergent results. See text for details. (Modified from Oliveri et al., 2000.)

lesions (Theoret, Haque, and Pascual-Leone, 2001) or prefrontal cortical lesions (Robertson et al., 2001; Mottaghy et al., in press) using the long-lasting effects of 1 Hz rTMS (Chen et al., 1997).

Lesions in subcortical brain areas cannot be mimicked by rTMS in the same fashion. In such instances, borrowing a patient's illness—that is, comparing the effects of transient disruption of cortical function in normal subjects and in patients with focal lesions in the basal ganglia or with degenerative basal ganglia diseases—might be the only means of approaching the questions. The use of implanted depth electrodes in the thalamus, globus pallidus, or subthalamic nucleus for the treatment of patients with Parkinson's disease or essential tremor provides a further opportunity to study cortico-subcortical interaction in vivo in the humans by borrowing patients' illnesses (Ashby and Rothwell, 2000). It is possible to use the implanted depth electrode to record brain activity during various motor or cognitive tasks, as also can be done in epileptic patients to localize the seizure focus. Furthermore, the effects of deep-brain stimulation on cortical excitability can be studied by comparing the effects of TMS to the motor cortex when the deep-brain stimulator is on or off (Chen et al., 2001). Chen et al. have shown that in Parkinsonian patients with depth electrodes implanted into the globus pallidus internus, deep brain stimulation is associated with a significant shortening of the silent period evoked by TMS of the ipsilateral motor cortex, whereas other measures of intracortical or corticospinal excitability were not changed. With a similar approach, it should be possible to compare the effects of TMS (single pulse or repetitive) on cognitive functions depending on the status of basal ganglia activation via implanted electrodes. Because a stimulus can be applied at a specific point in time through the implanted depth electrode, and the interval between the deep-brain stimulus and the TMS varied systematically, it will be possible to conduct chronometric studies of such cortico-subcortical interactions during motor and cognitive tasks.

THERAPEUTIC TMS

It is not our aim to present TMS as a therapeutic tool in neurology or psychiatry. Nevertheless, the possibility of modulating cortical excitability does indeed offer the possibility of applying TMS to normalize cortical excitability externally (to decrease it or increase it depending on the underlying dysfunction) and of assessing possible therapeutic benefits. The potential behavioral benefits of paradoxical lesion effects (see chapter 6) might have therapeutic significance. In this context, work has been done in depression, schizophrenia, obsessive-compulsive disorder, posttraumatic stress disorders, catatonia, Parkinson's disease, focal dystonia, tic disorders, myoclonus, and epilepsy (Paulus et al., 1999; George and Belmaker, 2000; Pascual-Leone et al., 2001). However, most of this work is preliminary and often has proved difficult to reproduce. It is actually unlikely that effects of TMS that may last sufficiently long to have a therapeutic significance for any neuropsychiatric disorder via the direct modulation of cortical excitability or even primary trans-synaptic effects of TMS (Pascual-Leone et al., 1998). TMS effects that are sustained enough to harbor a clinical therapeutic significance must be mediated by a cascade of neurophysiologic and neurochemical effects, including expression of early genes and eventual protein transcription. Such mechanisms of action are still unknown, and assessment of clinical significance of therapeutic TMS, even for medication-refractory depression, the area in which most studies have been conducted, requires multicenter clinical trials that have not been completed.

CONVERGING METHODOLOGIES: A MEETING OF MIND'S MAPS

MULTIDIMENSIONAL MAPPING

TMS, for all its virtues, is only one technique, and the map of the mind it provides comes from within the problem space presented in figure 1.1. It is not enough. To understand any cognitive function adequately, it is necessary to have the maps of brain function taken from within the problem spaces covered by other techniques. Generation of these maps needs other techniques to corroborate evidence or to ask different questions, and the researcher needs to use different techniques in conjunction with TMS to allow a view of one map through the coordinates of another. The combination of TMS with other techniques is just beginning, but what has been done so far has been useful in guiding and verifying the localization of TMS (Bohning et al., 1997, 1998, 1999; Fox et al., 1997; Paus et al., 1997, 1998; Paus and Wolforth, 1998; Paus, 1999; Bohning, 2000) and in generating hypotheses about the secondary loci of stimulation. The combination of these techniques and of TMS with EEG also has been driven by the desire to ask what these other techniques can tell us about TMS. What still awaits exploration are the many ways in which TMS can inform these other techniques. To see the brain through the different kinds of maps available adds other constraints on the interpretations of the results, and to apply these constraints requires knowledge of the shortcomings as well as the advantages of the techniques being combined.

All experimenters bring assumptions and expectations to the analysis of their results, and both can sometimes acquire the status of truths. A good example is often seen in brain-imaging experiments that obtain task-specific activations in two or more cortical or subcortical areas. If one of the areas is a sensory area and the second area is the parietal cortex or the frontal cortex, the interpretation is usually that the higher area in some way "modulated" the lower area. The evidence for these kinds of conclusions, however, is slim, and there are many historical warnings against attributing the physiology of apparently complex functions to the supposedly smarter areas in the brain. One classic example is that of illusory contours, which were so self-evidently a higher-order function of the brain that they were called "cognitive contours" and thus allocated a place in the inferotemporal cortex. We now know that the neural machinery required for the perception of illusory contours exists in V2 (Peterhans and von der Heydt, 1988) and V1 (Grosof, Shapley, and Hawken, 1993). Visual imagery provides another example of the increasing intelligence of the sensory cortex (Kosslyn et al., 1999). Imagination naturally was attributed to higher visual areas, but the combination of PET and rTMS has been able to establish necessary activity in area V1. Many other examples abound, and we have discussed some of them in previous chapters. Properties of sensory cortical areas are sufficient to explain priming of simple (Maljkovic and Nakayama, 1994, 1996; Walsh et al., 2000; Campana, Cowey, and Walsh, 2002) and complex objects (Bar and Biederman, 1999)—a function traditionally attributed to the parietal and frontal cortices. Working memory for stimulus attributes (Martin-Elkins, George, and Horel, 1989; Bisley and Pasternak, 2000) has now been shown to rely critically on visual areas such as V4 and V5/MT, not on the prefrontal cortex alone. The lesson here is that following a brain map made from surveying the brain with only one technique will contain as many blind alleys as clear highways.

TMS AND BRAIN IMAGING

We have seen already how TMS can be combined with EEG, PET, and fMRI, but we are at the very beginning of this story. Since Stallings et al. (1995) showed off-line TMS dose-related changes in perfusion of the prefrontal cortex, TMS and PET have been combined to locate the motor cortex (Wasserman et al., 1996), to investigate the cortical changes correlated with efficacy of rTMS in depression (George et al., 1996), to investigate cortico-cortical connectivity (Paus et al., 1997; Fox et al., 1997), and to show dose dependent changes in blood flow (Paus et al., 1998). TMS and MRI have been used to locate the site of activation by TMS (Roberts et al., 1997) and to correlate TMS behavioral effects with MRI activity (Kosslyn et al., 1999; Mottaghy et al., 2000). The idea of carrying fMRI and TMS simultaneously, however, initially was dismissed as impossible, mainly due to the fears of interactions between the brief but strong TMS field and the magnetic resonance scanner field. Bohning and colleagues, however, interpreted impossible as "difficult" and were the first to combine the two techniques simultaneously. They interleaved TMS and fMRI in a 1.5 Tesla scanner using a non–ferro magnetic figure-eight TMS coil. The TMS unit itself was stationed several meters from the scanner. The data were collected in cycles of rest-TMS-rest interleaved with acquisition of the magnetic resonance images, and the onset of TMS and EPI cycles was set to allow the effects of the TMS to dissipate before the RF pulse. This experiment successfully showed increased BOLD signal during TMS subcycles compared to rest and the activity was in the motor cortex, directly beneath the point of contact with the stimulating coil. Auditory cortex activity was also seen in response to the sound of the TMS pulses. Bohning et al. (1997) also have mapped the magnetic fields produced by TMS (not to be confused with the induced electric fields) and have ventured that combining stimulation with two coils strategically positioned to focus their peak field might reach areas that otherwise would be difficult to stimulate sufficiently. To our knowledge, this combination has not been tried in an experimental setting.

The information traffic between TMS and imaging is two way. Imaging can suggest times and places to stimulate in virtual-lesion experiments, and TMS can return new times, places, and interactions. The two techniques also can elucidate each other's mechanisms. We have detailed some of the imaging experiments aimed at investigating TMS, but Waldvogel et al. (2000) have asked the question, What is being recorded in fMRI studies—excitation or inhibition? To answer this question, they gave subjects a go/no-go task, measured TMS motor responses in each of the conditions, and found, as they expected, that MEPs were reduced for between 200 and 500 msec after the no-go signal relative to the go signal. They then carried out an event-related fMRI study while the subject carried out the same task and compared go versus no-go activity in the pre-SMA and the primary motor cortex. The anterior region was active in both response modes, but there was a significant decrease in BOLD signal in the motor cortex specifically related to the no-go trials. There was no deactivation of the motor cortex (the meaning of this is a separate issue), but simply a decreased change from rest. Waldvogel et al. concluded that inhibition is a metabollically more efficient process than excitation and that the signal seen in fMRI studies is therefore likely to reflect excitation.

TMS AND EEG

In chapter 1, we presented an empirical problem space to try to encapsulate the complementarity of the various techniques available and the significance of the differences between correlative and interference techniques. The complementary nature of TMS and EEG is a case of special interest to neurocognitive experimentation because both techniques rely on a high level of temporal resolution. However, neither the pulse width of magnetic stimulation nor the sampling rate of EEG recording captures the functional resolution of the two methods. As we have seen (cf. figure 3.16), a TMS effect can operate on any part of the waveform recorded with EEG, and there is little correspondence to be expected between the significant times of divergence of EEG signals or time to peak amplitude and the optimal times for TMS interference during a task (Ashbridge, Walsh, and Cowey, 1997; Walsh and Cowey, 1998, 2000). Ilmoniemi and colleagues (1997) combined TMS and EEG on-line (see chapter 3), but there is much to be gained by combining TMS and EEG off-line. The method involves using the distal application of TMS (chapter 4) at low frequencies to produce a medium-term change in behavioral performance and comparing EEG recordings taken before and after TMS. The development of this method requires attention to the heating effects of TMS pulses on electrodes (see Roth et al., 1992). Some tasks that already yield reliable TMS and ERP effects but that have not been used to compare the information across techniques are visual search (Luck and Hillyard, 1994; Ashbridge, Walsh, and Cowey, 1997), motion discrimination (Walsh et al., 1998; Stewart et al., 1999; Neville and Bavelier, 2000), priming (Rugg and Allen, 2000; Campana, Cowey, and Walsh, 2002), mathematical cognition (Dehaene, 1996; Göbel, personal communication), language processing (King and Kutas, 1995; Stewart et al., 2000, 2001) and plasticity (Pascual-Leone and Torres, 1993; Cohen et al., 1997; Classen et al., 1998; Walsh et al., 1998, 1999; Bütefisch et al., 2000; Neville and Bavelier, 2000).

The first question that distal TMS/off-line EEG might address is the relationship between EEG activity and necessary processes. TMS at 1 Hz over, say, the occipital cortex may disrupt the ability to detect lateralized targets, a function associated with the P1 component (Hillyard, Teder-Sälejärvi, and Münte, 1998). The question of interest, then, would be whether the P1 component was changed in a performance-dependent manner. A similar adaptation of an ERP paradigm to examine the psychological refractory period (PRP) (Luck, 1998) would also yield to a TMS-ERP manipulation, again the question being whether the ERP-recorded P300 would be delayed, diminished, or otherwise disrupted in line with a change in behavioral performance if 1 Hz TMS were applied over the parietal cortex before presenting subjects with the PRP task.

The combination of TMS and ERPs also can be used to assess the comparative chronometries of the methods. Single-pulse TMS interference typically occurs earlier than ERP peaks. This has two advantages: TMS can be used to divide the broad temporal window that covers the rise to peak amplitude of a waveform, and the two techniques, by offering different chronometries, can be used to test different kinds of temporal hypotheses. As discussed earlier, many processes may be continuous or gradual in their evolution, and it may be an error to expect to be able to isolate a critical time in a given process, and a null result in a single-pulse TMS experiment designed to test the necessity of ERP recorded activity may indicate a temporally indivisible process (in terms of there being a single critical time of neural activity) rather than a nonnecessary process being recorded by the ERPs.

Temporal interactions between areas also can be studied in an ERP-TMS-ERP paradigm. Jing and Takigawa (2000) have measured EEG coherence following rTMS and have shown that the ERP components can be delayed by distal TMS and that connectivity patterns can be changed. Jing et al. (2001) applied 10 Hz TMS for 3 sec at 100% of motor threshold over the left frontal cortex. Subjects were then presented with an auditory oddball paradigm during which EEG was measured from fourteen channels (figure 9.1). The P200 component was delayed by approximately 10 msec over left and midparietal sites, and the P300 latency increased over the right frontal cortex by 22 msec and by 15–17 msec at other electrode sites. However, Jing et al. do not report any behavioral effects of rTMS on the ERPs, so the correlation between EEG and behavioral change still has to be made. Jing et al. also calculated directed coherences (DCOH), a measure of the direction of information transfer, and argue that rTMS changed the pattern of information transfer, principally between frontal and temporal areas. The behavioral significance of these changes has not been established, but the method is clearly tractable.

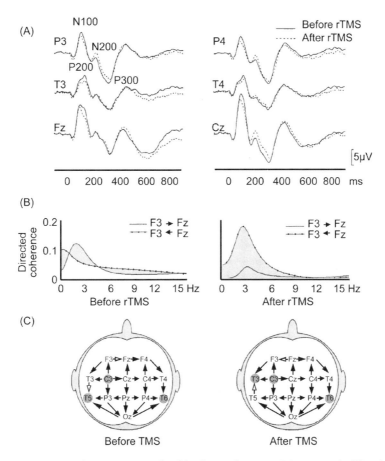

Figure 9.1   TMS and ERPs. An example of distal TMS changing ERPs measured off-line. (*A*) ERPs recorded before TMS are shown by the solid waveforms, and those recorded after TMS are shown by the dotted waveforms. An auditory tone was presented at time 0. (*B*) Measures of directed EEG coherence between two electrode sites before and after TMS, showing an increase in FZ-F3. (*C*) Inferred changes in functional information transfer between different electrode sites based on changes in directed coherence. (From Jing et al., 2001, with permission.)

TMS AND DRUGS

The combination of TMS with neuropharmacology is another area that has proved useful in studies of motor function but has not been applied to psychology. The measurement of drug effects typically is carried out using the paired-pulse paradigm with intracortical excitation measured before and sometime after administration of the drug. The major inhibitory transmitter in the mammalian central nervous system, γ-aminobutyric acid (GABA), enhances cortical inhibition and suppresses facilitation (Ziemann et al., 1995; Inghilleri et al., 1996; Ziemann, Rothwell, and Ridding, 1996). Correspondingly, blocking N-methyl-d-aspartate (NMDA) with glutamate antagonists increases paired-pulse inhibition and decreases facilitation (Liepert et al., 1997).

More complex manipulation of the neuropharmacology of learning has been combined with TMS. In a follow-up of the Classen et al. (1998) training experiment discussed in chapter 7, Bütefisch et al. (2000) conducted a study that replicated the effect and also tried to block the resulting plasticity by administering a drug (dextromethorphan) that blocks NMDA (necessary for long-term potentiation) or a GABA modulator that is known to block long-term potentiation (lorazepam). Bütefisch et al. administered the drugs before the subjects began the sequence of simple thumb movements. A control drug (lamotrigine) did not change the original training effect (Classen et al. 1998), but administration of lorazepam or dextromethorphan prevented the subsequent thumb movements from being elicited in the direction of training—the pattern of results was almost identical with the pretraining thumb movements (figure 9.2). These results can be taken as evidence that the plasticity observed in the studies discussed so far is due to NMDA inhibition of GABA activity to facilitate long-term potentiation. This does not solve the problem of why some actions and not others change the character of the MEP, and it will be interesting to see if the different time courses of the MEP changes and if their relationship to the behaviors performed can be parsed further by pharmacological manipulations.

TMS can produce chemical effects as well as be used to investigate them. Much of the work in this field has been motivated by clinical application

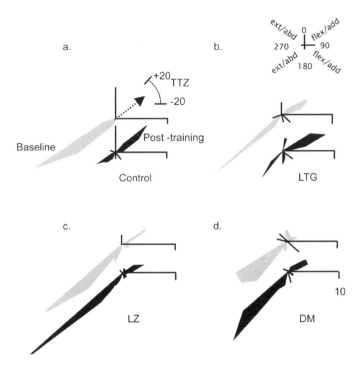

Figure 9.2   The effects of drugs on directional distribution of TMS-evoked movements in a single subject who has practiced a simple finger-flexion task (after Classen et al., 1998; see figure 7.12). Directions of TMS-evoked movements are shown in pairs of circular histograms for baseline (*upper, white plots*) and post-training (*lower, dark plots*). Frequencies are plotted on the same scale, and directions were binned in 10° steps. The mean training angle (*arrow*) and the target zone for the directed thumb movement (training target zone, TTZ) for control and the three drug conditions are shown in (*a*). The control group and a group taking lamotrigine (LTG, a drug that does not affect long-term potentiation) the direction of the post-training TMS-elicited thumb twitches were in the trained direction. In subjects who took lorazepam (LZ) or dextromethorphan (DM), both of which block long-term potentiation, the TMS-elicited thumb twitches were in the same direction as the baseline movements, not in the trained direction. (From Bütefisch et al., 2000, with permission.)

(Pridmore and Belmaker, 1999; George and Belmaker, 2000), but the outcomes point to clear applications in basic investigations. Hausmann et al. (2000) observed the effects of chronic rTMS on the expression of the immediate early gene c-fos (presumed to be an indicator of neural activation). Rats were given 20 Hz TMS for 10 sec at 75% of MagStim rapid output over fourteen days. The expression of c-fos was found to be increased in layer VI of the parietal cortex and also in the hippocampus. These selective effects are difficult to interpret because of the relatively large size of the coil with respect to the rats' heads. Nevertheless, the paradigms to advance this kind of work, which aims to provide a link between TMS and events at the cellular level, are being tested, and some work has attempted to extend this link to behavioral correlates of the TMS. Keck et al. (2000a), for example, have investigated the effects of rTMS (twenty trains of 20 Hz for 2.5 sec with an intertrain interval of 2 min at 130% motor threshold) on rats' responses in a forced swim test. The coil was a figure eight (57 mm outer diameter wings—again rather large relative to the rat) and was aimed at the left frontal cortex. The TMS-treated rats displayed improved coping strategies (defined as more attempts to get out of the water), when compared to the sham-treated control group, though there were no differences on an elevated-plus maze or changes in social behavior. However, measurements of release of corticotropin (ACTH) after exposure to the elevated-plus maze were significantly lower in the TMS group than in controls. It has been reported that rTMS can have neuroprotective effects (Post et al., 1999), selectively modulate the release of a range of biogenic amines (Keck et al., 2000b), and also increase expression of brain-derived neurotrophic factors (BDNF) and cholecystokinin (CCK) (Muller et al., 2000), but it remains to be seen how closely the link can be made between cellular effects of TMS and behavior. At the very least, this work should stimulate the further use of animal models in TMS.

TMS AND OTHER ANIMALS

TMS is most effective when targeting areas on the surface of the brain, and many areas are therefore out of reach in human cortex (for example, ventral visual areas). Monkeys, however, have less-convoluted brains, and areas that are buried ventrally or medially in the human brain are accessible on the surface of the macaque brain, so these animals present possibilities for other types of experiments. Developing TMS in monkeys in comparison with aspiration lesions, carries all the scientific advantages of TMS used in patient studies. It also can reduce the numbers of monkeys needed for a lesion experiment because the animals can be used as their own controls, needn't be sacrificed for histology, and can be compared with human subjects who have undergone exactly the same experimental procedures, thus strengthening and testing assumptions of homology. TMS on monkeys has been carried out mainly in studies of the motor cortex (e.g., Lemon, Muir, and Mantel, 1987; Amassian, Quirk, and Stewart, 1990; Edgeley et al., 1992; Flament, Hall, and Lemon, 1992), and the extension to cognitive studies will encounter several problems. The small size of a monkey's head will make anatomical images a necessity, and the thickness of the muscle over a monkey's skull may also present a problem. Monkeys also will need to be chair restrained for the delivery of TMS, but this can be done noninvasively (Cowey and Stoerig, 1995). The method most likely to succeed is the distal method of TMS (see figure 4.9), which will obviate the need to train monkeys to carry out tasks while receiving TMS. Further work also needs to be done on coil design for stimulation of monkey cortex because the induced electric field is decreased as a function of brain size (Weissman, Epstein, and Davey, 1992).

CONCLUSION

Everyone likes to prove himself or herself right, and we are unlikely to have written a book on new possibilities offered by a technique simply to change our minds at the end. But in writing this book, we have felt a deep sense of excitement generated by just how many possibilities are opened up by the virtual-lesion approach and also a sense of frustration that we have spent too much time writing a book when new experiments are staring us in the face. In discussing these experiments on learning, priming, cortical back projections, mathematical cognition, spatial attention, TMS and long-term potentiation, TMS and fMRI, TMS in monkeys, and many other aspects of neuropsychology, we have come to the conclusion that our very first claim in the book is correct after all: Cognitive neuropsychologists indeed have never had it so good.

References

Abdeen, M. A., and Stuchley, M. A. (1994). Modelling of magnetic stimulation of bent neurons: IEEE. *IEEE Transactions in Biomedical Engineering* 41: 1092–1095.

Afra, J., Mascia, A., Gerard, P., Meartens de Noordhout, A., and Schoenen, J. (1998). Interictal cortical excitability in migraine: A study using transcranial magnetic stimulation of motor and visual cortices. *Annals of Neurology* 44: 209–215.

Allen, K., and Rugg, M. D. (1997). An event-related potential study of explicit memory on tests of cued recall and recognition. *Neuropsychologia* 35: 387–397.

Amassian, V. E., Cracco, R. Q., Maccabee, P. J., Cracco, J. B., Rudell, A. P., and Eberle, L. (1989). Suppression of visual perception by magnetic coil stimulation of human occipital cortex. *Electroencephalography and Clinical Neurophysiology* 74: 458–462.

Amassian, V. E., Quirk, G. J., and Stewart, A. (1990). A comparison of corticospinal activation by magnetic coil and electrical stimulation of monkey motor cortex. *Electroencephalography and Clinical Neurophysiology* 77: 390–401.

Amassian, V. E., Somasundaram, M., Rothwell, J. C., Britton, T., Cracco, J. B., Cracco, R. Q., Maccabee, P. J., and Day, B. L. (1991). Paraesthesias are elicited by single pulse, magnetic coil stimulation of motor cortex in susceptible humans. *Brain* 114 (pt. 6): 2505–2520.

Amassian, V. E., Eberle, L., Maccabee, P. J., and Cracco, R. Q. (1992). Modeling magnetic coil excitation of human cerebral cortex with a peripheral nerve immersed in a brain shaped volume conductor: The significance of fiber-bending in excitation. *Electroencephalography and Clinical Neurophysiology* 85: 291–301.

Amassian, V. E., Cracco, R. Q., Maccabee, P. J., Cracco, J. B., Rudell, A. P., and Eberle, L. (1993a). Unmasking human visual perception with the magnetic coil and its relationship to hemispheric asymmetry. *Brain Research* 605: 312–316.

Amassian, V. E., Maccabee, P. J., Cracco, R. Q., Cracco, J. B., Rudell, A. P., and Eberle, L. (1993b). Measurement of information processing delays in human visual cortex with repetitive magnetic coil stimulation. *Brain Research* 605: 317–321.

Amassian, V. E., Maccabee, P. J., and Cracco, P. Q. (1994). The polarity of the induced electric field influences magnetic coil inhibition of human visual cortex: Implications for the site of excitation. *Electroencaphalography and Clinical Neurophysiology* 93: 21–26.

Amassian, V. E., Cracco, R. Q., Maccabee, P. J., Cracco, J. B., Rudell, A. P., and Eberle, L. (1998). Transcranial magnetic stimulation in study of the visual pathway. *Journal of Clinical Neurophysiology* 15: 288–304.

Arguin, M., Joanette, Y., and Cavanagh, P. (1990). Comparing the cerebral hemispheres on the speed of spatial shifts of visual attention: Evidence from serial search. *Neuropsychologia* 28: 733–736.

Arguin, M., Joanette, Y., and Cavanagh, P. (1993). Visual search for feature and conjunction targets with an attention deficit. *Journal of Cognitive Neuroscience* 5: 436–452.

Ashbridge, E., Walsh, V., and Cowey. A. (1997). Temporal aspects of visual search studied by transcranial magnetic stimulation. *Neuropsychologia* 35: 1121–1131.

Ashby, P., and Rothwell, J. C. (2000). Neurophysiologic aspects of deep brain stimulation. *Neurology* 55 (supp. 6): S17–S20.

———

Aurora, S. K., Ahmad, B. K., Welch, K. M., Bhardhwaj, P., and Ramadan, N. M. (1998). Transcranial magnetic stimulation confirms hyperexcitability of occipital cortex in migraine. *Neurology* 50: 1111–1114.

Bar, M., and Biederman, I. (1999). Localizing the cortical region mediating visual awareness of object identity. *Proceedings of the National Academy of Sciences* 96: 1790–1793.

Barbur, J., Watson, J. D. G., Frackowiak, R. S. J., and Zeki, S. M. (1993). Conscious visual perception without V1. *Brain* 116: 1293–1302.

Barbur, J., Wolf, J., and Lennie, P. (1998). Visual processing levels revealed by response latencies to changes in different visual attributes. *Proceedings of the Royal Society B* 265: 2321–2325.

Barbur, J., Wolf, J., and Lennie, P. (1999). The unseen color aftereffect of an unseen stimulus: Insight from blindsight into mechanisms of color afterimages. *Proceedings of the National Academy of Science, U.S.A.* 96: 11637–11641.

Barker, A. T. (1976). Determination of the distribution of conduction velocities in human nerve trunks. Ph.D. thesis, University of Sheffield.

Barker, A. T. (1991). An introduction to the basic principles of magnetic nerve stimulation. *Journal of Clinical Neurophysiology* 8: 26–37.

Barker, A. T. (1999). The history and basic principles of magnetic nerve stimulation. *Electroencephalography and Clinical Neurophysiology* supp. 51: 3–21.

Barker, A. T., Freeston, I. L. (1985). Magnetic stimulation of the human brain. *Journal of Physiology* (London) 369: 3P (abstract).

Barker, A. T., Jalinous, R., and Freeston, I. L. (1985). Non-invasive magnetic stimulation of the human motor cortex. *Lancet* 1: 1106–1107.

Barker, A. T., Freeston, I. L., Jalinous, R., and Jarratt, J. A. (1986). Clinical evaluation of conduction time measurements in central motor pathways using magnetic stimulation of the human brain. *Lancet* 1: 1325–1326.

———

233

Barker, A. T., Freeston, I. L., Jalinous, R., and Jarratt, J. A. (1987). Magnetic stimulation of the human brain and peripheral nervous system: An introduction and the results of an initial clinical evaluation. *Neurosurgery* 20: 100–109.

Barlow, H. B., Kohn, H. L., and Walsh, E. G. (1947). Visual sensations aroused by magnetic fields. *American Journal of Physiology* 148: 372–375.

Bartolomeo, P., Bachoud-Levi, A. C., Degos, J. D., and Boller, F. (1998). Disruption of residual reading capacity in a pure alexic patient after a mirror-image right-hemispheric lesion. *Neurology* 286–288.

Bartres-Faz, D., Pujol, J., Deus, J., Tormos, J. M., Keenan, J. P., and Pascual-Leone, A. (Submitted). Is the speech arrest induced by repetitive transcranial magnetic stimulation due to disruption of the motor cortex?

Baseler, H., Morland, A. B., and Wandell, B. (1999). Topographic organization of human visual areas in the absence of input from primary visual cortex. *Journal of Neuroscience* 19: 2619–2627.

Beckers, G., and Zeki, S. (1995). The consequences of inactivating areas V1 and V5 on visual motion perception. *Brain* 118 (pt. 1): 49–60.

Beer, B. (1902). Über das Auftretten einer objectiven Lichtempfindung in magnetischen Felde. *Klinische Wochenzeitschrift* 15: 108–109.

Berardelli, A., Inghilleri, M., Polidori, L., Priori, A., Mercuri, B., and Manfredi, M. (1994). Effects of transcranial magnetic stimulation on single and sequential arm movements. *Experimental Brain Research* 98: 501–506.

Berardelli, A., Inghilleri, M., Rothwell, J. C., Romeo, S., Curra, A., Gilio, F., Modugno, N., and Manfredi, M. (1998). Facilitation of muscle evoked responses after repetitive cortical stimulation in man. *Experimental Brain Research* 122: 79–84.

Bichot, N. P., Rao, S. C., and Schall, J. D. (in press). Continuous processing in macaque frontal cortex during visual search. *Neuropsychologia.*

Bickford, R. G., and Fremming, B. D. (1965). Neural stimulation by pulsed magnetic fields in animals and man. *Digest of the 6th International Conference on Medical Electronics and Biological Engineering* (Tokyo): 6.

Bisiach, E., and Vallar, G. (1988). Hemineglect in humans. In *Handbook of Neuropsychology,* F. Boller and J. Grafman (eds.). Amsterdam: Elsevier Science, pp. 195–222.

Bisiach, E., Geminiani, G., Berti, A., and Rusconi, M. L. (1990). Perceptual and premotor factors of unilateral neglect. *Neurology* 40: 1278–1281.

Bisiach, E., Rusconi, M. L., Peretti, V. A., and Vallar, G. (1994). Challenging current accounts of unilateral neglect. *Neuropsychologia* 32: 1431–1434.

Bisiach, E., Pizzamiglio, L., Nico, D., and Antonucci, G. (1996). Beyond unilateral neglect. *Brain* 119: 851–857.

Bisley, J. W., and Pasternak, T. (2000). The multiple roles of visual cortical areas MT/MST in remembering the direction of visual motion. *Cerebral Cortex* 10: 1053–1065.

Blakemore, S.-J., and Frith, C. D. (2000). Functional neuroimaging in studies of schizophrenia. In *Brain Mapping: The Disorders,* J. C. Mazziotta, A. W. Toga, and R. S. J. Frackowiak (eds.). New York: Academic Press, pp. 523–544.

Bogdahn, U. (1998). *Transcranial Doppler Sonography.* London: Blackwell Science.

Bohning, D. E. (2000). Introduction and overview of TMS physics. In *Transcranial Magnetic Stimulation in Neuropsychiatry,* M. S. George and R. H. Bellmaker (eds.). Washington, D.C.: American Psychiatric Press, pp. 13–44.

Bohning, D. E., Pecheny, A. P., Epstein, C. M., Vincent, D. J., Dannels, W. R., and George, M. S. (1997). Mapping transcranial magnetic stimulation (TMS) fields in vivo with MRI. *Neuroreport* 8: 2535–2538.

Bohning, D. E., Shastri, A., Nahas, Z., Lorberbaum, J. P., Andersen, S. W., Dannels, W. R., Haxthausen, E. U., Vincent, D. J., and George, M. S. (1998). Echoplanar BOLD fMRI of brain activation induced by concurrent transcranial magnetic stimulation. *Investigative Radiology* 33: 336–340.

Bohning, D. E., Shastri, A., Blumenthal, K. M., Nahas, Z., Lorberbaum, J., Roberts, D., Teneback, C., Vincent, D. J., and George, M. S. (1999). A combined TMS/fMRI study of intensity-dependent TMS over motor cortex. *Biological Psychiatry* 45: 385–394.

Boroojerdi, B., Bushara, K. O., Corwell, B., Immisch, I., Battaglia, F., Muellbacher, W., and Cohen, L. (2000a). Enhanced excitability of the human visual cortex induced by short term light deprivation. *Cerebral Cortex* 10: 529–534.

Boroojerdi, B., Prager, A., Muellbacher, W., and Cohen, L. (2000b). Reduction of human visual cortex excitability using 1-Hz transcranial magnetic stimulation. *Neurology* 54: 1529–1531.

Bowers, D., and Heilman, K. M. (1980). Material-specific hemispheric activation. *Neuropsychologia* 18: 309–319.

Brasil-Neto, J. P., Cohen, L. G., Panizza, M., Nilsson, J., Roth, B. J., and Hallett, M. (1992a). Optimal focal transcranial magnetic activation of the human motor cortex: Effects of coil orientation, shape of the induced current pulse, and stimulus intensity. *Journal of Clinical Neurophysiology* 9: 132–136.

Brasil-Neto, J. P., Cohen, L. G., Pascual-Leone, A., Jabir, F. K., Wall, R. T., and Hallett, M. (1992b). Rapid reversible modulation of human motor outputs after transient deafferentation of the forearm: A study with transcranial magnetic stimulation. *Neurology* 42: 1302–1306.

Brasil-Neto, J. P., McShane, L. M., Fuhr, P., Hallett, M., and Cohen, L. G. (1992c). Topographic mapping of the human motor cortex with magnetic stimulation: Factors affecting accuracy and reproducibility. *Electroencephalography and Clinical Neurophysiology* 85: 9–16.

Brasil-Neto, J. P., Valls-Sole, J., Pascual-Leone, A., Cammarota, A., Amassian, V. E., Cracco, R., Maccabee, P., Cracco, J., Hallett, M., and Cohen, L. G. (1993). Rapid modulation of human cortical motor outputs following ischaemic nerve block. *Brain* 116 (pt. 3): 511–525.

———

Bravo, M. J., and Nakayama, K. (1992). The role of attention in different visual search tasks. *Perception and Psychophysics* 51: 465–472.

Buckner, R. L., Bandettini, P. O., O'Craven, K. M., Savoy, R. L., Petersen, S. E., Raichle, M. E., and Rosen, B. R. (1996). Detection of cortical activation during averaged single trials of a cognitive task using functional magnetic resonance imaging. *Proceedings of the National Academy of Sciences, U.S.A.* 93: 14878–14883.

Bullier, J. (2003). Cortical connections and functional interactions between visual cortical areas. In *Neuropsychology of Vision,* M. Fahle (ed.). Oxford: Oxford University Press, pp. 151–179.

Burnstine, T. H., Lesser, R. P., Hart, J., Uematsu, S., Zinreich, S. J., Krauss, G. L., Fisher, R. S., Vining, E. P., and Gordon, B. (1990). Characterization of the basal temporal language area in patients with left temporal lobe epilepsy. *Neurology* 40: 966–970.

Bütefisch, C. M., Davis, B. C., Wise, S. P., Sawaki, L., Kopylev, L., Classen, J., and Cohen, L. G. (2000). Mechanisms of use dependent plasticity in the human motor cortex. *Proceedings of the National Academy of Science, U.S.A.* 97: 3661–3665.

Butter, C. M. (1968). The effects of discrimination training on pattern equivalence in monkeys with inferotemporal and lateral striate lesions. *Neuropsychologia* 6: 27–40.

Butter, C. M. (1969). Impairments in selective attention to visual stimuli in monkeys with inferotemporal and lateral striate lesions. *Brain Research* 12: 374–383.

Butter, C. M. (1972). Detection of masked patterns in monkeys with inferotemporal, striate or dorsolateral frontal lesions. *Neuropsychologia* 10: 241–243.

Butterworth, B. (1999). *The Mathematical Brain.* Chapham, Kent: MacMillan.

Campana, G., Cowey, A., and Walsh, V. (2002). Visual priming of motion direction depends on area V5/MT but not on striate or parietal cortex. *Cerebral Cortex* 12: 663–669.

Caramia, M. D., Palmieri, M. G., Giacomini, P., Iani, C., Dally, I., and Silvestrini, M. (2000). Ipsilateral activation of the unaffected motor cortex in patients with hemiparetic stroke. *Clinical Neurophysiology* 111: 1990–1996.

Carlesimo, G. A., Fadda, L., Sabbadini, M., and Caltagirone, C. (1994). Visual repetition priming for words relies on access to the visual input lexicon: Evidence from a dyslexic patient. *Neuropsychologia* 32: 1089–1100.

Catano, A., Houa, M., Caroyer, J. M., Ducarne, H., and Noel, P. (1996). Magnetic transcranial stimulation in acute stroke: Early excitation threshold and functional prognosis. *Electroencephalography and Clinical Neurophysiology* 101: 233–239.

Catano, A., Houa, M., and Noel, P. (1997). Magnetic transcranial stimulation: Dissociation of excitatory and inhibitory mechanisms in acute strokes. *Electroencephalography and Clinical Neurophysiology* 105: 29–36.

Cavada, C., and Goldman-Rakic, P. S. (1993). Multiple visual areas in the posterior parietal cortex of primates. *Progress in Brain Research* 95: 123–137.

Celebrini, S., Thorpe, S., Trotter, Y., and Imbert, M. (1993). Dynamics of orientation coding in area V1 of the awake primate. *Visual Neuroscience* 10: 811–825.

Chen, R., Classen, J., Gerloff, C., Celnik, P., Wassermann, E. M., Hallett, M., and Cohen, L. G. (1997a). Depression of motor cortex excitability by low-frequency transcranial magnetic stimulation. *Neurology* 48: 1398–1403.

Chen, R., Wassermann, E. M., Canos, M., and Hallett, M. (1997b). Impaired inhibition in writer's cramp during voluntary muscle activation. *Neurology* 49: 1054–1059.

Chen, R., Garg, R. R., Lozano, A. M., and Lang, A. E. (2001). Effects of internal globus pallidus stimulation on motor cortex excitability. *Neurology* 27: 716–723.

Chiappa, K. H., Cros, D., Day, B. L., Fang, J., MacDonnell, R., and Mavroudakis, N. (1991). Magnetic stimulation of the human motor cortex: Ipsilateral and contralateral facilitation effects. *Electroencephalography and Clinical Neurophysiology* supp. 43: 186–201.

Chochon, F., Cohen, L., van de Moortele, P.-F., and Dehaene, S. (1999). Differential contributions of the left and right inferior parietal lobules to number processing. *Journal of Cognitive Neuroscience* 11: 617–630.

Chomsky, N. (1967). *Current Issues in Linguistic Theory*. The Hague: Mouton.

Chronicle, E. P., and Mulleners, W. (1996). Visual system dysfunction in migraine: A review of clinical and psychophysical findings. *Cephalalgia* 16: 525–535.

Classen, J., Liepert, J., Wise, S. P., Hallett, M., and Cohen, L. G. (1998). Rapid plasticity of human cortical movement representation induced by practice. *Journal of Neurophysiology* 79: 1117–1123.

Claus, D., Weis, M., Jahnke, U., Plewe, A., and Brunholzl, C. (1992). Corticospinal conduction studied with magnetic double stimulation in the intact human. *Journal of the Neurological Sciences* 111: 180–188.

Cohen, J. D., Romero, R. D., Servanschreiber, D., and Farah, M. J. (1994). Mechanisms of spatial attention: The relation of macrostructure to microstructure in parietal neglect. *Journal of Cognitive Neuroscience* 6: 377–387.

Cohen, L. G., Bandinelli, S., Findley, T. W., and Hallett, M. (1991a). Motor reorganization after upper limb amputation in man: A study with focal magnetic stimulation. *Brain* 114 (pt. 1B): 615–627.

Cohen, L. G., Bandinelli, S., Sato, S., Kufta, C., and Hallett, M. (1991b). Attenuation in detection of somatosensory stimuli by transcranial magnetic stimulation. *Electroencephalography and Clinical Neurophysiology* 81: 366–376.

Cohen, L. G., Meer, J., Tarkka, I., Bierner, S., Leiderman, D. B., Dubinsky, R. M., Sanes, J. N., Jabbari, B., Branscum, B., and Hallett, M. (1991c). Congenital mirror movements: Abnormal organization of motor pathways in two patients. *Brain* 114: 381–403.

Cohen, L. G., Topka, H., Cole, R. A., and Hallett, M. (1991d). Leg paresthesias induced by magnetic brain stimulation in patients with thoracic spinal cord injury. *Neurology* 41: 1283–1288.

Cohen, L. G., Celnik, P., Pascual-Leone, A., Corwell, B., Falz, L., Dambrosia, J., Honda, M., Sadato, N., Gerloff, C., Catala, M. D., and Hallett, M. (1997). Functional relevance of cross-modal plasticity in blind humans. *Nature* 389: 180–183.

Coles, M. G. H., Smid, H. G., Scheffers, M. K., and Otten, L. J. (1995). Mental chronometry and the study of human information processing. In *Electrophysiology of Mind: Event-Related Brain Potentials and Cognition,* M. D. Rugg and M. G. H. Coles (eds.). Oxford: Oxford University Press, pp. 86–131.

Collin, N. G., Cowey, A., Latto, R., and Marzi, C. (1982). The role of frontal eye fields and superior colliculi in visual search and non-visual search in rhesus monkeys. *Behavioural Brain Research* 4: 177–193.

Corbetta, M., Miezin, F. M., Dobmeyer, S., Shulman, G. L., and Petersen, S. E. (1991). Selective and divided attention during visual discriminations of shape, color, and speed: Functional anatomy by positron emission tomography. *Journal of Neuroscience* 11: 2383–2402.

Corbetta, M., Miezin, F. M., Shulman, G. L., and Petersen, S. E. (1993). A PET study of visual spatial attention. *Journal of Neuroscience* 13: 1202–1226.

Corbetta, M., Shulman, G. L., Miezin, F. M., and Petersen, S. E. (1995). Superior parietal cortex activation during spatial attention shifts and visual feature conjunction. *Science* 270: 802–805.

Corthout, E., Uttl, B., Walsh, V., Hallett, M., and Cowey, A. (1999a). Timing of activity in early visual cortex as revealed by transcranial magnetic stimulation. *Neuroreport* 10: 1–4.

Corthout, E., Uttl, B., Ziemann, U., Cowey, A., and Hallett, M. (1999b). Two periods of processing in the (circum)striate visual cortex as revealed by transcranial magnetic stimulation. *Neuropsychologia* 37: 137–145.

Corthout, E., Uttl, B., Walsh, V., Hallet, M., and Cowey, A. (2000). Plasticity revealed by transcranial magnetic stimulation of early visual cortex. *Neuroreport* 11: 1565–1569.

Coslett, H. B., and Monsul, N. (1994). Reading with the right hemisphere: Evidence from transcranial magnetic stimulation. *Brain and Language* 46: 198–211.

Cowell, S. F., Egan, G. F., Code, C., Harasty, J., and Watson, J. D. G. (2000). The functional neuroanatomy of simple calculation and number repetition: A parametric PET activation study. *NeuroImage* 12: 565–573.

Cowey, A. (1964). The projection of the retina onto the striate and the prestriate cortex in the squirrel monkey, *Saimiri sciurens. Journal of Neurophysiology* 27: 366–393.

Cowey, A., and Gross, C. G. (1970). Effects of foveal prestriate and inferotemporal lesions on visual discrimination by rhesus monkeys. *Experimental Brain Research* 11: 128–144.

Cowey, A., and Stoerig, P. (1991). The neurobiology of blindsight. *Trends in Neuroscience* 14: 140–145.

Cowey, A., and Stoerig, P. (1995). Blindsight in monkeys. *Nature* 373: 247–249.

Cowey, A., and Walsh, V. (2000). Magnetically induced phosphenes in sighted, blind, and blindsighted observers. *Neuroreport* 11: 3269–3273.

Cowey, A., and Walsh, V. (2001). Tickling the brain. *Progress in Brain Research*. 134: 411–425.

Crick, F., and Koch, C. (1998). Consciousness and neuroscience. *Cerebral Cortex* 8: 97–103.

Critchley, M. (1953). *The Parietal Lobes.* New York: Hafner.

Damasio, H., and Damasio, A. R. (1989). *Lesion Analysis in Neuropsychology*. Oxford: Oxford University Press.

Damasio, H., Grabowski, T., Frank, R., Galaburda, A. M., and Damasio, A. R. (1994). The return of Phineas Gage: Clues about the brain from the skull of a famous patient. *Science* 264: 1102–1105.

d'Arsonval, A. (1896). Dispositifs pour la mesure des courants alternatifs de toutes frequences. *CR Societe Biologique* (Paris) (May 2): 450–451.

Day, B. L., Thompson, P. D., Dick, J. P., Nakashima, K., and Marsden, C. D. (1987). Different sites of action of electrical and magnetic stimulation of the human brain. *Neuroscience Letters* 75: 101–106.

Day, B. L., Dressler, D., Maertens de Noordhout, A., Marsden, C. D., Nakashima, K., Rothwell, J. C., and Thompson, C. D. (1989a). Electric and magnetic stimulation of the human motor cortex: Surface EMG and single motor unit responses. *Journal of Physiology* 412: 449–473.

Day, B. L., Rothwell, J. C., Thompson, P. D., Maertens de Noordhout, A., Nakashima, K., Shannon, K., and Marsden, C. D. (1989b). Delay in the execution of voluntary movement by electrical or magnetic brain stimulation in intact man: Evidence for the storage of motor programs in the brain. *Brain* 112 (pt. 3): 649–663.

Day, P. (1999). *The Philosopher's Tree: A Selection of Michael Faraday's Writings.* Bristol, U.K.: Institute of Physics.

Dehaene, S. (1996). The organization of brain activation in number comparisons: Event-related potentials and the additive factors methods. *Journal of Cognitive Neuroscience* 8: 47–68.

Dehaene, S. (1997). *The Number Sense.* London: Penguin.

Dehaene, S., Tzourio, N., Fraka, V., Raynaud, L., Cohene, L., Mehler, J., and Mazoyer, B. (1996). Cerebral activations during number multiplication and comparison: A PET study. *Neuropsychologia* 34: 1097–1196.

Delgado, J. M. R. (1965). *Evolution of Physical Control of the Brain.* New York: American Museum of Natural History.

Delgado, J. M. R. (1980). Control físico de la mente: Hacia una sociedad psicocivilizada. 3rd ed. Madrid: Espasa Calpe.

Desimone, R., and Duncan, J. (1995). Neural mechanisms of selective visual attention. *Annual Review of Neuroscience* 18: 193–222.

Desmurget, M., Epstein, C. M., Turner, R. S., Prablanc, C., Alexander, G. E., and Grafton, S. T. (1999). Role of the posterior parietal cortex in updating reaching movements to a visual target [see comments]. *Nature Neuroscience* 2: 563–567.

Donders, F. C. (1969). On the speed of mental processes. In *Attention and Performance II*. W. G. Koster (ed.). Amsterdam: North-Holland, pp. 412–431.

Dorf, R. C. (1986). *Modern Control Systems*. 5th ed. Reading, Mass.: Addison Wesley.

Duncan, J., and Humphreys, G. W. (1989). Visual search and stimulus similarity. *Psychological Review* 96: 433–458.

Dunlap, K. (1911). Visual sensations from the alternating magnetic field. *Science* 33: 68–71.

Edgeley, S. A., Eyre, J. A., Lemon, R. N., and Miller, S. (1992). Direct and indirect activation of the corticospinal tract by electromagnetic and elecrical stimulation of the scalp in the macaque monkey. *Journal of Physiology* 425: 310–320.

Ellison, A., Battelli, L., Walsh, V., and Cowey, A. (Submitted). The effects of expectation on corticocortical interactions in visual search: A TMS study.

Ellison, A., Rushworth, M. F. S., and Walsh, V. (Submitted). Parsing the contribution of the parietal cortex in visual search: Visual, spatial, and response requirements.

Epstein, C., and Zangaladze, A. (1996). Magnetic coil suppression of extrafoveal visual perception using disappearance targets. *Journal of Clinical Neurophysiology* 13: 242–246.

Epstein, C. M., Lah, J. J., Meador, K., Weissman, J. D., Gaitan, L. E., and Dihenia, B. (1996). Optimum stimulus parameters for lateralized suppression of speech with magnetic brain stimulation. *Neurology* 47: 1590–1593.

Epstein, C., Verson, R., and Zangaladze, A. (1996). Magnetic coil suppression of visual perception at an extracalcarine site. *Journal of Clinical Neurophysiology* 13: 247–252.

Epstein, C. M., Meador, K. J., Loring, D. W., Wright, R. J., Weissman, J. D., Sheppard, S., Lah, J. J., Puhalovich, F., Gaitan, L., and Davey, K. R. (1999). Localization and characterization of speech arrest during transcranial magnetic stimulation. *Clinical Neurophysiology* 110: 1073–1079.

Eyre, J. A., Miller, S., and Ramesh, V. (1991). Constancy of central conduction delays during development in man: Investigation of motor and somatosensory pathways. *Journal of Physiology* 434: 441–452.

Fadiga, L., Fogassi, L., Pavesi, G., and Rizzolatti, G. (1995). Motor facilitation during action observation: A magnetic stimulation study. *Journal of Neurophysiology* 73: 2608–2611.

Fadiga, L., Buccino, G., Craighero, L., Fogassi, L., Gallese, V., and Pavesi, G. (1999). Corticospinal excitability is specifically modulated by motor imagery: A magnetic stimulation study. *Neuropsychologia* 37: 147–158.

Farah, M., and Wallace, M. (1993). "What" and "where" in visual attention: Evidence from the neglect syndrome. In *Unilateral Neglect: Clinical and Experimental Studies*. I. H. Robertson and J. C. Marshal (eds.). Hillsdale, N. J.: Erlbaum, pp. 17–35.

Ferrier, D. (1875). Experiments on the brains of monkeys. *Philosophical Transactions of the Royal Society of London* 165: 433.

Ferrier, D. (1876). *The Functions of the Brain*. London: Dawsons.

Ferrier, D. (1890). *The Croonian Lecturer on Cerebral Localization*.

Fierro, B., Brighina, F., Oliveri, M., Piazza, A., La Bua, V., Buffa, D., and Bisiach, E. (2000). Contralateral neglect induced by right posterior parietal rTMS in healthy subjects. *Neuroreport* 11: 1519–1521.

Flament, D., Hall, E. J., and Lemon, R. J. (1992). The development of corticomotorneuronal projections investigated using magnetic brain stimulation in the infant macaque. *Journal of Physiology* 447: 755–768.

Flitman, S. S., Grafman, J., Wassermann, E. M., Cooper, V., O'Grady, J., Pascual-Leone, A., and Hallett, M. (1998). Linguistic processing during repetitive transcranial magnetic stimulation. *Neurology* 50: 175–181.

Fox, P., Ingham, R., George, M. S., Mayberg, H. S., Ingham, J., Roby, J., Martin, C., and Jerabek, P. (1997). Imaging human intra-cerebral connectivity by PET during TMS. *Neuroreport* 8: 2787–2791.

Friedman-Hill, S. R., Robertson, L. C., and Treisman, A. (1995). Parietal contributions to visual feature binding: Evidence from a patient with bilateral lesions. *Science* 269: 853–855.

Gabrieli, J. D. E., Fleischman, D. A., Keane, M. M., Reminger, S. L., and Morrell, F. (1995). Double dissociation between memory systems underlying explicit and implicit memory in the human brain. *Psychological Science* 6: 76–82.

Galbraith, J. K. (1990). *A Short History of Financial Euphoria*. London: Penguin.

Ganis, G., Keenan, J. P., Kosslyn, S. M., and Pascual-Leone, A. (2000). Transcranial magnetic stimulation of primary motor cortex affects mental rotation. *Cerebral Cortex* 10: 175–180.

Garnham, C. W., Barker, A. T., and Freeston, I. L. (1995). Measurement of the activating function of magnetic stimulation using combined electrical and magnetic stimuli. *Journal of Medical Engineering and Technology* 19: 57–61.

Gauld, A. (1992). *A History of Hypnotism*. Cambridge: Cambridge University Press.

Gazzaniga, M., Bogen, J. E., and Sperry, R. E. (1962). Some functional effects of sectioning the cerebral commisures. *Proceedings of the National Academy of Science* 245: 947–952.

Geddes, L. A. (1991). History of magnetic stimulation of the nervous system. *Journal of Clinical Neurophysiology* 8: 3–9.

George, M. S., and Belmaker, R. H. (eds.). (2000). *Transcranial Magnetic Stimulation in Neuropsychiatry*. Washington D.C.: American Psychiatric Press.

George, M. S., Wassermann, E. M., Williams, W. A., Callahan, A., Ketter, T. A., Basser, P., Hallett, M., and Post, R. M. (1995). Daily repetitive transcranial magnetic stimulation (rTMS) improves mood in depression. *Neuroreport* 6: 1853–1856.

George, M. S., Wassermann, E. M., Williams, W. A., Steppel, J., Pascual-Leone, A., Basser, P., Hallett, M., and Post, R. M. (1996). Changes in mood and hormone levels after rapid-rate transcranial magnetic stimulation (rTMS) of the prefrontal cortex. *Journal of Neuropsychiatry and Clinical Neurosciences* 8: 172–180.

Gerloff, C., Corwell, B., Chen, R., Hallett, M., and Cohen, L. G. (1997). Stimulation over the human supplementary motor area interferes with the organization of future elements in complex motor sequences. *Brain* 120 (pt. 9): 1587–1602.

Gilbert, W. (1600). *De Magnete.* New York: Dover.

Göbel, S., Walsh, V., and Rushworth, M. (2001). The mental number line: A TMS study. *NeuroImage* 14: 1278–1289.

Goldman-Rakic, P. S. (1998). The prefrontal landscape: Implications of functional architecture for understanding human mentation and the central executive. In *The Prefrontal Cortex,* A. C. Roberts, T. W. Robbins, and L. Weiskrantz (eds.). Oxford: Oxford University Press, pp. 121–153.

Grabowsa, T. J., and Damasio, A. R. (2000). Investigating language with functional neuroimaging. In *Brain Mapping: The Systems,* A. W. Toga and J. C. Mazziotta (eds.). New York: Academic, pp. 425–446.

Grafman, J., Pascual-Leone, A., Alway, D., Nichelli, P., Gomez-Tortosa, E., and Hallett, M. (1994). Induction of a recall deficit by rapid rate transcranial magnetic stimulation. *Neuroreport* 5: 1157–1160.

Grosof, D. H., Shapley, R. M., and Hawken, M. J. (1993). Macaque V1 neurons can signal illusory contours. *Nature* 365: 550–552.

Gross, C. G. (1978). Inferior temporal lesions do not impair discrimination of rotated patterns in monkeys. *Journal of Comparative and Physiological Psychology* 92: 1095–1109.

Gross, C. G., Cowey, A., and Manning, F. J. (1971). Further analysis of visual discrimination deficits following foveal prestriate and inferotemporal lesions in monkeys. *Journal of Comparative and Physiological Psychology* 76: 1–7.

Hadjikhani, N., Liu, A. K., Dale, A. M., Cavanagh, P., and Tootell, R. B. H (1998). Retinotopy and color sensitivity in human visual cortical area V8. *Nature Neuroscience* 1: 235–241.

Haenny, P. E., and Schiller, P. H. (1988). State dependent activity in monkey visual cortex. I. Single cell activity in V1 and V4 on visual tasks. *Experimental Brain Research* 69: 225–244.

Haenny, P. E., Maunsell, J. H. R., and Schiller, P. H. (1988). State dependent activity in monkey visual cortex. II. Retinal and extraretinal factors in V4. *Experimental Brain Research* 69: 245–259.

Haggard, P., and Magno, E. (1999). Localising awareness of action with transcranial magnetic stimulation. *Experimental Brain Research* 127: 102–107.

Hall, E. J., Flament, D., Fraser, C., and Lemon, R. N. (1990). Non-invasive brain stimulation reveals reorganised cortical outputs in amputees. *Neuroscience Letters* 116: 379–386.

Hallett, M. (1995). Transcranial magnetic stimulation: Negative effects. *Advances in Neurology* 67: 107–113.

Hallett, M. (1996). Transcranial magnetic stimulation: A useful tool for clinical neurophysiology [editorial, comment]. *Annals of Neurology* 40: 344–345.

Hallett, M., Luders, H. O., and Marsden, C. D. (eds.). (1995). *Negative Motor Phenomena*. Philadelphia: Lippincott-Raven.

Hausmann, A., Weis, C., Marksteiner, J., Hinterhuber, H., and Humpel, C. (2000). Chronic repetitive transcranial magnetic stimulation enhances c-fos in the parietal cortex and hippocampus. *Molecular Brain Research* 76: 355–362.

———

Heinen, F., Fietzek, U. M., Berweck, S., Hufschnidt, A., Deuschl, G., and Korinthenberg, R. (1998). The fast corticospinal system and motor performance in children: Conduction precedes skill. *Journal of Paediatric Neurology* supp. 19: 217–221.

Hess, C. W., Mills, K. R., and Murray, N. M. F. (1986). Magnetic stimulation of the human brain: Facilitation of motor responses by voluntary contraction of the ipsilateral and contra-lateral muscles with additional observation on an amputee. *Neuroscience Letters* 71: 235–240.

Hilgetag, C. C., Kotter, R., and Young, M. P. (1999). Interhemispheric competition of sub-cortical structures is a crucial mechanism in paradoxical lesion effects and spatial neglect. *Progress in Brain Research* 121: 121–141.

Hilgetag, C. C., Theoret, H., and Pascual-Leone, A. (2001). Enhancement of visual spatial attention ipsilateral to TMS-induced "virtual lesions" of human parietal cortex. *Nature Neuroscience* 4: 953–957.

Hill, A. C., Davey, N. J., and Kennard, C. (2000). Current orientation induced by magnetic stimulation influences a cognitive task. *Neuroreport* 11: 1–3.

Hillyard, S. A., Teder-Sälejärvi, W. A., and Münte, T. F. (1998). Temporal dynamics of early perceptual processing. *Current Opinion in Neurobiology* 8: 202–210.

Hinde, R. A., Rowell, T. E., and Spencer-Booth, Y. (1964). Behaviour of socially living rhesus monkeys in their first six months. *Proceedings of the Zoological Society* 143: 609–648.

Hodgkin, A. L., and Huxley, A. F. (1939). Action potentials recorded from inside a nerve fibre. *Journal of Physiology* (London) 144: 710–711.

Holliday, I. E., Anderson, S. J., and Harding, G. F. A. (1997). Magnetoencephalographic evidence for non-geniculate visual input to human area V5. *Neuropsychologia* 35: 1139–1146.

Hopfinger, J. B., and Mangun, G. R. (1998). Reflexive attention modulates processing of visual stimuli in human extrastriate cortex. *Psychological Science* 9: 441–447.

Horel, J. A. (1996). Perception, learning, and identification studied with reversible suppression of cortical visual areas in monkeys. *Behavioural Brain Research* 76: 199–214.

Hotson, J. R., and Anand, S. (1999). The selectivity and timing of motion processing in human temporo-parieto-occipital and occipital cortex: A transcranial magnetic stimulation study. *Neuropsychologia* 37: 169–179.

Hotson, J. R., Braun, D., Herzberg, W., and Boman, D. (1994). Transcranial magnetic stimulation of extrastriate cortex degrades human motion direction discrimination. *Vision Research* 34: 2115–2123.

Hubel, D. H., and Wiesel, T. N. (1968). Receptive fields and functional architecture of monkey striate cortex. *Journal of Physiology* 195: 215–243.

Hupe, J.-M., Chouvet, G., and Bullier, J. (1999a). Spatial and temporal parameters of cortical inactivation by GABA. *Journal of Neuroscience Methods* 86: 129–144.

Hupe, J. M., James, A. A., Payne, B. R., Lomber, S. G., Girard, P., and Bullier, J. (1999b). Cortical feedback improves discrimination between figure and background by V1, V2, and V3 neurons. *Nature* 394: 784–787.

Hupe, J. M., James, A. C., Girard, P., Lomber, S. G., Payne, B. R., and Bullier, J. (2001). Feedback connections act on the early part of the responses in monkey visual cortex. *Journal of Neurophysiology* 85: 134–145.

Ilmoniemi, R. J., Virtanen, J., Ruohonen, J., Karhu, J., Aronen, H. J., Naatanen, R., and Katila, T. (1997). Neuronal responses to magnetic stimulation reveal cortical reactivity and connectivity. *Neuroreport* 8: 3537–3540.

Ingvar, D. (1983). Serial aspects of language and speech relative to prefrontal cortical activity. *Human Neurobiology* 2: 77–89.

Iwai, E., and Mishkin, M. (1969). Further evidence on the locus of the visual area in the temporal lobe of the monkey. *Experimental Neurology* 25: 585–594.

Izumi, S., Takase, M., Arita, M., Masakado, Y., Kimura, A., and Chino, N. (1997). Transcranial magnetic stimulation–induced changes in EEG and responses recorded from the scalp of healthy humans. *Electroencephalography and Clinical Neurophysiology* 103: 319–322.

Jalinous, R. (1991). Technical and practical aspects of magnetic nerve stimulation. *Journal of Clinical Neurophysiology* 8: 10–25.

Jalinous, R. (1995). *Guide to Magnetic Stimulation*. Whitland, Wales: Magstim.

James, F. A. (1993). *The Correspondence of Michael Faraday*. London: Institute of Electrical Engineers.

Jennum, P., Friberg, L., Fuglsang-Frederiksen, A., and Dam, M. (1994). Speech localization using repetitive transcranial magnetic stimulation. *Neurology* 44: 269–273.

Jennum, P., Winkel, H., and Fuglsang-Frederiksen, A. (1995). Repetitive magnetic stimulation and motor evoked potentials. *Electroencephalography and Clinical Neurophysiology* 97: 96–101.

Jing, H., and Takigawa, M. (2000). Observation of EEG coherence after repetitive transcranial magnetic stimulation. *Clinical Neurophysiology* 111: 1620–1631.

Jing, H., Takigawa, M., Hamada, K., Okamura, H., Kawaika, Y., Yonezawa, T., and Fukuzako, H. (2001). Effects of high frequency repetitive transcranial magnetic stimulation on P300 event-related potentials. *Clinical Neurophysiology* 112: 304–313.

Kammer, T. (1999). Phosphenes and transient scotomas induced by magnetic stimulation of the occipital lobe: Their topographic relationship. *Neuropsychologia* 37: 191–198.

Kammer, T., and Nusseck, H. G. (1998). Are recognition deficits following occipital lobe TMS explained by raised detection thresholds? *Neuropsychologia* 36: 1161–1166.

Kammer, T., Beck, S., Thielscher, A., Laubis-Herrman, U., and Topka, H. (2001). Motor thresholds in humans: A transcranial magnetic stimulation study comparing different pulse waveforms, current directions, and stimulator types. *Clinical Neurophysiology* 112: 250–258.

Kapur, N. (1996). Paradoxical functional facilitation in brain-behaviour research: A critical review. *Brain* 119: 1775–1790.

Kastner, S., Demmer, I., and Ziemann, U. (1998). Transient visual field defects induced by transcranial magnetic stimulation over human occipital pole. *Experimental Brain Research* 118: 19–26.

Kawamichi, H., Kikuchi, Y., Endo, H., Takeda, T., and Yoshizowa, S. (1998). Temporal structure of implicit motor imagery in viual hand shape discrimination as revealed by MEG. *Neuroreport* 9: 1127–1132.

Keck, M. E., Engelman, M., Muller, M. B., Henniger, M. S. H., Hermann, B., Rupprecht, R., Neumann, I. D., Toschi, N., Landgraf, R., and Post, A. (2000a). Repetitive transcranial magnetic stimulation induces active coping strategies and attenuates the neuroendocrine stress response in rats. *Journal of Psychiatric Research* 34: 265–276.

Keck, M. E., Sillaber, I., Ebner, K., Welt, T., Toschi, N., Kaehler, S. T., Singewald, N., Philippu, A., Elbel, G. K., Wotjak, C. T., Holsboer, F., Landgraf, R., and Engelmann, M. (2000b). Acute transcranial magnetic stimulation of frontal brain regions selectively modulates the release of vasopressin, biogenic amines, and amino acids in the rat brain. *European Journal of Neuroscience* 12: 3713–3720.

Kew, J. J., Ridding, M. C., Rothwell, J. C., Passingham, R. E., Leigh, P. N., Sooriakumaran, S., Frackowiak, R. S., and Brooks, D. J. (1994). Reorganization of cortical blood flow and transcranial magnetic stimulation maps in human subjects after upper limb amputation. *Journal of Neurophysiology* 72: 2517–2524.

Kimura, D. (1993). *Neuromotor Mechanisms in Human Communication*. New York: Clarendon.

Kimura, D., and Archibald, Y. (1974). Motor functions of the left hemisphere. *Brain* 97: 337–350.

King, J. W., and Kutas, M. (1995). Who did what and when? Using word and clause-related ERPs to monitor working memory usage in reading. *Journal of Cognitive Neuroscience* 7: 378–397.

———

Kinsbourne, M. (1977). Hemi-neglect and hemisphere rivalry. *Advances in Neurology* 18: 41–49.

Konogaya, Y., Mano, Y., and Konogaya, M. (1990). Magnetic stimulation study in mirror movements. *Journal of Neurology* 237: 107–109.

Kossyln, S. M. (1980). *Image and Mind*. Cambridge, Mass.: MIT Press.

Kosslyn, S. M. (1988). Aspects of a cognitive neuroscience of mental imagery. *Science* 240: 1621–1626.

Kosslyn, S. M. (1994). *Images and the Brain*. Cambridge, Mass.: MIT Press.

Kosslyn, S. M., Alpert, N. M., Thompson, W. L., Maljkovic, V., Weise, S. B., Chabris, C. F., Hamilton, S. E., Rauch, S. L., and Buonanno, F. S. (1993a). Visual mental imagery activates topographically organized visual cortex: PET investigations. *Journal of Cognitive Neuroscience* 5: 263–287.

Kosslyn, S. M., Daly, P. F., McPeek, R. M., Alpert, N. M., Kennedy, D. N., and Caviness, V. S. J. (1993b). Using locations to store shape: An indirect effect of a lesion. *Cerebral Cortex* 3: 567–582.

Kosslyn, S. M., Pascual-Leone, A., Felician, O., Camposano, S., Keenan, J. P., Thompson, W. L., Ganis, G., Sukel, K. E., and Alpert, N. M. (1999). The role of area 17 in visual imagery: Convergent evidence from PET and rTMS [see comments]. *Science* 284: 167–170. [Published erratum appears in *Science* 284 (1999):197.]

Krings, T., Buchbinder, B. R., Butler, W. E., Chiappa, K. H., Jiang, H. J., Cosgrove, G. R., and Rosen, B. R. (1997a). Functional magnetic resonance imaging and transcranial magnetic stimulation: Complementary approaches in the evaluation of cortical motor function. *Neurology* 48: 1406–1416.

Krings, T., Buchbinder, B. R., Butler, W. E., Chiappa, K. H., Jiang, H. J., Rosen, B. R., and Cosgrove, G. R. (1997b). Stereotactic transcranial magnetic stimulation: Correlation with direct electrical cortical stimulation. *Neurosurgery* 41: 1319–1325.

Krings, T., Naujokat, C., and von Keyserlingk, D. G. (1998). Representation of cortical motor function as revealed by stereotactic transcranial magnetic stimulation. *Electroencephalography and Clinical Neurophysiology* 109: 85–93.

Kuhn, T. (1970). *The Structure of Scientific Revolutions*. 2d ed. Chicago: University of Chicago Press.

Kujirai, T., Caramia, M. D., Rothwell, J. C., Day, B. L., Thompson, B. D., and Ferbert, A. (1993). Cortico-cortical inhibition in human motor cortex. *Journal of Physiology* (London) 471: 501–520.

Lawrence, D. G., and Hopkins, D. A. (1976). The development of motor control in the rhesus monkey: Evidence concerning the role of corticomotoneuronal connections. *Brain* 99: 235–254.

Lawrence, D. G., and Kuypers, H. G. J. M. (1968). The functional organisation of the motor system. 1. The effects of bilateral pyramidal lesions. *Brain* 91: 1–14.

Lemon, R. N., Muir, R. B., and Mantel, G. W. H. (1987). The effects upon the activity of hand and forearm muscles of intracortical stimulation in the vicinity of corticomotor neurons in the conscious monkey. *Experimental Brain Research* 66: 621–637.

Lemon, R. N., Johansson, R. S., and Westling, G. (1995). Corticospinal control during reach, grasp, and precision lift in man. *Journal of Neuroscience* 15: 6145–6156.

Li, J., Hotson, J. R., and Boman, D. K. (1994). Enhancement of anticipatory smooth eye movement velocities with magnetic stimulation. *Investigative Ophthalmology and Vision Science* 35: 1349.

Libet, B., Gleason, C. A., Wright, E. W., and Pearl, D. K. (1983). Tone of conscious intention to act in relation to onset of cerebral activity (readiness-potential). *Brain* 106: 623–642.

Liepert, J., Teggenthoff, M., and Malin, J.-P. (1995). Changes of cortical motor area size during immobilization. *Electroencephalography and Clinical Neurophysiology* 97: 382–386.

Livingstone, M. S., and Hubel, D. H. (1984). Anatomy and physiology of a color system in the primate visual system. *Journal of Neuroscience* 4: 309–356.

Lomber, S. (1999). The advantages and limitations of permanent or reversible deactivation techniques in the assessment of neural function. *Journal of Neuroscience Methods* 86: 109–118.

Lomber, S. G., and Payne, B. R. (1996). Removal of two halves restores the whole: Reversal of visual hemineglect during bilateral cortical or collicular inactivation in the cat. *Visual Neuroscience* 13: 1143–1156.

Lomber, S. G., and Payne, B. R. (1999). Assessment of neural function with reversible deactivation methods. *Journal of Neuroscience Methods* 86: 105–108.

Lomber, S. G., Payne, B. R., and Horel, J. A. (1999). The cryoloop: An adaptable reversible cooling deactivation method for behavioural or electrophysiological assessment of neural function. *Journal of Neuroscience Methods* 86: 179–194.

Lovsund, P., Oberg, P. A., Nilsson, S. E., and Reuter, T. (1980). Magnetophosphenes: A quantitative analysis of thresholds. *Medical and Biological Engineering and Computing* 18: 326–334.

Luck, S. (1998). Sources of dual-task interference: Evidence from human electrophysiology. *Psychological Science* 9: 223–227.

Luck, S. J., and Hillyard, S. A. (1994). Electrophysiological correlates of feature analysis during visual search. *Psychophysiology* 31: 291–308.

Lueck, C. J., Zeki, S., Friston, K. J., Deiber, M. P., Cope, P., Cunningham, V. J., Lammertsma, A. A., Kennard, C., and Frackowiak, R. S. (1994). The colour centre in the cerebral cortex of man. *Nature* 340: 386–389.

Lynch, A. C. (1989). Silvanus Thompson: Teacher, researcher, historian. *IEEE Proceedings* 136 (pt. A, no. 6): 306–312.

Maccabee, P. J., Amassian, V. A., Cracco, R. Q., Zemon, V., Rudell, A., and Eberle, L. (1989). Suppression of chromatic and achromatic letter perception by magnetic coil stimulation of human visual cortex. *Society for Neuroscience Abstracts* 15: 121.

Maccabee, P. J., Eberle, L., Amassian, V. E., Cracco, R. Q., Rudell, A., and Jayachandra, M. (1990). Spatial distribution of the electric field induced in volume by round and figure "8" magnetic coils: Relevance to activation of sensory nerve fibres. *Electroencephalography and Clinical Neurophysiology* 76: 131–141.

Maccabee, P. J., Amassian, V. E., Cracco, R. Q., Cracco, J. B., Rudell, A. P., Eberle, L. P., and Zemon, V. (1991). Magnetic coil stimulation of human visual cortex: Studies of perception. In *Magnetic Motor Stimulation: Basic Principles and Clinical Experience,* W. J. Levy, R. Q. Cracco, A. T. Barker, and J. Rothwell (eds.). Amsterdam: Elsevier Science, pp. 111–120.

Maccabee, P. J., Amassian, V. E., Eberle, L. P., and Cracco, R. Q. (1993). Magnetic coil stimulation of straight and bent amphibian and mammalian peripheral nerve in vitro: Locus of excitation. *Journal of Physiology* (London) 460: 201–219.

Mackay, G., and Dunlop, J. C. (1899). The cerebral lesions in a case of complete acquired colour-blindness. *Scottish Medical and Surgical Journal* 5: 503–512.

Maeda, F., and Pascual-Leone, A. (In press). Transcranial magnetic stimulation: Studying the neurophysiology of psychiatric disorders and their treatment. *Psychopharmacology*.

Maeda, F., Keenan, J. P., and Pascual-Leone, A. (2000). Interhemispheric asymmetry of motor cortical excitability in major depression as measured by transcranial magnetic stimulation. *British Journal of Psychiatry* 177: 169–173.

Maeda, F., Keenan, J. P., Tormos, J. M., Topka, H., and Pascual-Leone, A. (2000). Modulation of corticospinal excitability by repetitive transcranial magnetic stimulation. *Clinical Neurophysiology* 111: 800–805.

Magnussen, S. (2000). Low level memory processes in vision. *Trends in Neuroscience* 23: 247–251.

Magnussen, S., and Greenlee, M. W. (1999). The psychophysics of perceptual memory. *Psychological Research* 62: 81–92.

Magnusson, C. E., and Stevens, H. C. (1911). Visual sensations induced by the changes in the strength of a magnetic field. *American Journal of Physiology* 29: 124–136.

Magnusson, C. E., and Stevens, H. C. (1914). Visual sensation caused by a magnetic field. *Philosophy Magazine* 28: 188–207.

Maljkovic, V., and Nakayama, K. (1994). Priming of pop-out. I. Role of features. *Memory and Cognition* 22: 657–672.

Maljkovic, V., and Nakayama, K. (1996). Priming of pop-out. II. The role of position. *Perception and Psychophysics* 58: 977–991.

Malpeli, J. G. (1999). Reversible inactivation of subcortical sites by drug injection. *Journal of Neuroscience Methods* 86: 119–128.

Mangun, G. R., and Hillyard, S. A. (1988). Spatial gradients of visual attention: Behavioural and electrophysiological evidence. *Electroencephalography and Clinical Neurophysiology* 70: 417–428.

Marangolo, P., Di Pace, E., Rafal, R., and Scabini, D. (1998). Effects of parietal lesions in humans on color and location priming. *Journal of Cognitive Neuroscience* 10: 704–716.

Marg, E. (1991). Magnetostimulation of vision: Direct noninvasive stimulation of the retina and the visual brain. *Optometry and Visual Science* 68: 427–440.

Marg, E., and Rudiak, D. (1994). Phosphenes induced by magnetic stimulation over the occipital brain: Description and probably site of stimulation. *Optometry and Vision Science* 71: 301–311.

Marr, D. (1982). *Vision.* San Francisco: Freeman.

Martin, J. H., and Chez, G. (1999). Pharmacological inactivation in the analysis of the central control of movement. *Journal of Neuroscience Methods* 86: 1145–1160.

———

Martin-Elkins, C. L., George, P., and Horel, J. A. (1989). Retention deficits produced in monkeys with reversible cold lesions in the prestriate cortex. *Behavioural Brain Research* 32: 219–230.

Marzi, C. A., Miniussi, C., Maravita, A., Bertolasi, L., Zanette, G., Rothwell, J. C., and Sanes, J. N. (1998). Transcranial magnetic stimulation selectively impairs interhemispheric transfer of visuo-motor information in humans. *Experimental Brain Research* 118: 435–438.

Masur, H., Papke, K., and Oberwittler, C. (1993). Suppression of visual perception by transcranial magnetic stimulation: Experimental findings in healthy subjects and patients with optic neuritis. *Electroencephalography and Clinical Neurophysiology* 86: 259–267.

Mathis, J., de Quervain, D., and Hess, C. W. (1998). Dependence of the transcranially induced silent period on the "instruction set" and the individual reaction time. *Electroencephalography and Clinical Neurophysiology* 109: 426–435.

Maunsell, J. H. R., and Gibson, J. R. (1992). Visual response latencies in striate cortex of the macaque monkey. *Journal of Neurophysiology* 68: 1332–1344.

McBride, E. R., and Rothstein, A. L. (1979). Mental and physical practice and the learning and retention of open and closed skills. *Perceptual and Motor Skills* 49: 359–365.

McCarthy, R. A., and Warrington, E. K., (1990). *Cognitive Neuropsychology: A Clinical Introduction*. San Diego, London: Academic.

McCourt, M. E., and Jewell, G. (1999). Visuospatial attention in line bisection: Stimulus modulation of pseudoneglect. *Neuropsychologia* 37: 843–855.

McGuire, E. A., Frackowiak, R. S. J., and Frith, C. D. (1997). Recalling routes around London: Activation of the right hippocampus in taxi drivers. *Journal of Neuroscience* 17: 7103–7110.

McHenry, I. C. (1969). *Garrison's History of Neurology*. Springfield, Ill.: Charles C. Thomas.

McLeod, P., Heywood, C. A., Driver, J., and Zihl, J. (1989). Selective deficits of visual search in moving displays after extrastriate damage. *Nature* 339: 466–467.

McRobbie, D., and Foster, M. A. (1984). Thresholds for biological effect of time-varying magnetic fields. *Clinical Physiology and Physiological Measures* 2: 67–78.

Mendoza, D. W., and Wichman, H. (1978). "Inner" darts: Effects of mental practice on performance of dart throwing. *Perceptual and Motor Skills* 47: 1195–1199.

Merton, P. A., and Morton, H. B. (1980). Stimulation of the cerebral cortex in the intact human subject (letter). *Nature* 285: 227.

Mesulam, M. M. (1981). A cortical network for directed attention and unilateral neglect. *Annals of Neurology* 4: 309–325.

Meyer, B.-U., Diehl, R., Steinmetz, H., Britten, T. C., and Benecke, R. (1991). Magnetic stimuli applied over motor and visual cortex: Influence of coil position and field polarity on motor responses, phosphenes, and eye movements. *Electroencephalography and Clinical Neurophysiology* supp. 43: 121–134.

Meyer, D. E., Osman, A. M., Irwin, D. E., and Yantis, S. (1988). Modern mental chronometry. *Biological Psychology* 26: 3–67.

Michaels, C. F., and Turvey, M. T. (1979). Central sources of visual masking: Indexing structures supporting seeing at a single, brief glance. *Psychological Research* 41: 1–61.

Miller, J. O. (1988). Discrete and continuous models of human information processing: Theoretical distinctions and empirical results. *Acta Psychologia* 67: 191–257.

Miller, M. B., Fendrich, R., Eliassen, J. C., Demirel, S., and Gazzaniga, M. S. (1996). Transcranial magnetic stimulation: Delays in visual suppression due to luminance changes. *Neuroreport* 7: 1740–1744.

Mills, K. R. (1999). *Magnetic Stimulation of the Human Nervous System*. Oxford: Oxford University Press.

Milner, A. D., and Goodale, M. A. (1995). *The Visual Brain in Action*. Oxford: Oxford University Press.

———

Milner, B. (1966). Amnesia following operation on the temporal lobes. In *Amnesia,* C. W. M. Whitty and O. L. Zangwill (eds.). London: Botterworths, pp. 109–133.

Milner, B., Squire, L. R., and Kandel, E. R. (1998). Cognitive neuroscience and the study of memory. *Neuron* 20: 445–468.

Moore, C. J., and Price, C. J. (1999). Three distinct ventral occipitotemporal regions for reading and object naming. *NeuroImage* 10: 181–192.

Moran, J., and Desimone, R. (1985). Selective attention gates visual processing in the extrastriate cortex. *Science* 229: 782–784.

Morioka, T., Mizushima, A., Yamamoto, T., Tobimatsu, S., Matsumoto, S., Hasuo, K., Fujii, K., and Fukui, M. (1995a). Functional mapping of the sensorimotor cortex: Combined use of magnetoencephalography, functional MRI, and motor evoked potentials. *Neuroradiology* 37: 526–530.

Morioka, T., Yamamoto, T., Mizushima, A., Tombimatsu, S., Shigeto, H., Hasuo, K., Nishio, S., Fujii, K., and Fukui, M. (1995b). Comparison of magnetoencephalography, functional MRI, and motor evoked potentials in the localization of the sensory-motor cortex. *Neurological Research* 17: 361–367.

Mottaghy, F. M., Hungs, M., Brugmann, M., Sparing, R., Boroojerdi, B., Foltys, H., Huber, W., and Topper, R. (1999). Facilitation of picture naming after repetitive transcranial magnetic stimulation. *Neurology* 53: 1806–1812.

Mottaghy, F. M., Krause, B. J., Kemna, L. J., Topper, R., Tellmann, L., Beu, M., Pascual-Leone, A., and Muller-Gartner, H. W. (2000). Modulation of the neuronal circuitry subserving working memory in healthy human subjects by repetitive transcranial magnetic stimulation. *Neuroscience Letters* 280: 167–170.

Mottaghy, F. M., Gangitano, M., Sparing, R., Krause, B. J., and Pascual-Leone, A. (2002). Segregation of areas related to visual working memory in the prefrontal cortex revealed by rTMS. *Cerebral Cortex* 12: 369–375.

Moutoussis, K., and Zeki, S. (1997). A direct demonstration of perceptual asynchrony in vision. *Proceedings of the Royal Society of London B* 264: 393–399.

Moyer, R., and Bayer, R. (1976). Mental comparison and the symbolic distance effect. *Cognitive Psychology* 8: 228–246.

Muellbacher, W., Artner, C., and Mamoli, B. (1999). The role of the intact hemisphere in recovery of midline muscles after recent monohemispheric stroke. *Journal of Neurology* 246: 250–256.

Mulleners, W. M., Chronicle, F. P., Palmer, J. E., Koehler, P. J., and Vredeveld, J.-W. (2001). Visual cortex excitability in migraine with and without aura. *Headache* 41: 565–572.

Muller, M. B., Toschi, N., Kresse, A. E., Post, A., and Keck, M. E. (2000). Long-term repetitive transcranial magnetic stimulation increases the expression of brain-derived neurotrophic factor and cholecystokinin mRNA, but not neuropeptide tyrosine mRNA in specific areas of rat brain. *Neuropsychopharmacology* 23: 205–215.

Muri, R. M., Hess, C. W., and Meienberg, O. (1991). Transcranial stimulation of the human frontal eye field by magnetic pulses. *Experimental Brain Research* 86: 219–223.

Muri, R. M., Rosler, K. M., and Hess, C. W. (1994). Influence of transcranial magnetic stimulation on the execution of memorised sequences of saccades in man. *Experimental Brain Research* 101: 521–524.

Muri, R. M., Rivaud, S., Vermersch, A. I., Leger, J. M., and Pierrot-Deseilligny, C. (1995). Effects of transcranial magnetic stimulation over the region of the supplementary motor area during sequences of memory-guided saccades. *Experimental Brain Research* 104: 163–166.

Muri, R. M., Vermersch, A. I., Rivaud, S., Gaymard, B., and Pierrot-Deseilligny, C. (1996). Effects of single-pulse transcranial magnetic stimulation over the prefrontal and posterior parietal cortices during memory-guided saccades in humans. *Journal of Neurophysiology* 76: 2102–2106.

Muri, R. M., Rivaud, S., Gaymard, B., Ploner, C. J., Vermersch, A. I., Hess, C. W., and Pierrot-Deseilligny, C. (1999). Role of the prefrontal cortex in the control of express saccades: A transcranial magnetic stimulation study. *Neuropsychologia* 37: 199–206.

Muri, R. M., Gaymard, B., Rivaud, S., Vermersch, A. I., Hess, C. W., and Pierrot-Deseilligny, C. (2000). Hemispheric asymmetry in cortical control of memory-guided saccades: A transcranial magnetic stimulation study. *Neuropsychologia* 38: 1105–1111.

Murray, N. M. F. (1992). The clinical usefulness of magnetic cortical stimulation. *Electroencephalography and Clinical Neurophysiology* 85: 81–85.

Nagarajan, S. S., Durand, D. M., and Warman, E. N. (1993). Effects of induced electric fields on finite neuronal structures: A simulation study. *IEEE Transactions in Biomedical Engineering* 40: 1175–1188.

Neville, H., and Bavelier, D. (2000). Specificity and plasticity in neurocognitive development in humans. In *The New Cognitive Neurosciences,* M. S. Gazzaniga (ed.). Cambridge, Mass.: MIT Press, pp. 83–98.

Niehaus, L., Rorricht, S., Scholz, U., and Meyer, B.-U. (1999). Hemodynamic response to repetitive magnetic stimulation of the motor and visual cortex. *Electroencephalography and Clinical Neurophysiology* supp. 51: 41–47.

Nowak, L. G., Munk, M. H., Girard, P., and Bullier, J. (1995). Visual latencies in areas V1 and V2 of the macaque monkey. *Visual Neuroscience* 12: 371–384.

Ojemann, G. (1983). Brain organization for language from the perspective of electrical stimulation mapping. *Behavioural and Brain Sciences* 6: 189–230.

Ojemann, G., and Mateer, C. (1979). Human language cortex: Localization of memory, syntax, and sequential motor-phoneme identification systems. *Science* 1401–1403.

Oliveri, M., Rossini, P. M., Pasqualetti, P., Traversa, R., Cicinelli, P., Palmieri, M. G., Tomaiuolo, F., and Caltagirone, C. (1999a). Interhemispheric asymmetries in the perception of unimanual and bimanual cutaneous stimuli: A study using transcranial magnetic stimulation. *Brain* 122 (pt. 9): 1721–1729.

Oliveri, M., Rossini, P. M., Traversa, R., Cicinelli, P., Filippi, M. M., Pasqualetti, P., Tomaiuolo, F., and Caltagirone, C. (1999b). Left frontal transcranial magnetic stimulation reduces contralesional extinction in patients with unilateral right brain damage. *Brain* 122 (pt. 9): 1731–1739.

O'Breathnach, U., and Walsh, V. (1999). Jump starting the brain. *Current Biology* 9: R184–185.

Oliveri, M., Caltagirone, C., Filippi, M. M., Traversa, R., Cicinelli, P., Pasqualetti, P., and Rossini, P. M. (2000). Paired transcranial magnetic stimulation protocols reveal a pattern of inhibition and facilitation in the human parietal cortex. *Journal of Physiology* 529: 461–468.

Oster, G. (1970). Phosphenes. *Scientific American* 222: 82–87.

Oyachi, H., and Ohtsuka, K. (1995). Transcranial magnetic stimulation of the posterior parietal cortex degrades accuracy of memory-guided saccades in humans. *Investigative Ophthalmology and Visual Science* 36: 1441–1449.

Pardo, J., Pardo, P., Janer, K., and Raichle, M. (1990). The anterior cingulate cortex mediates processing selection in the stroop attentional conflict paradigm. *Proceedings of the National Academy of Science U.S.A.* 87: 256–259.

Pascual-Leone, A., and Torres, F. (1993). Plasticity of the sensorimotor cortex representation of the reading finger in Braille readers. *Brain* 116 (pt. 1): 39–52.

Pascual-Leone, A., and Walsh, V. (2001). Fast back projections from the motion area to the primary visual area necessary for visual awareness. *Science* 292: 510–512.

Pascual-Leone, A., Brasil-Neto, J., Valls-Solé, J., Cohen, L. G., and Hallett, M. (1991a). Simple reaction time to focal transcranial magnetic stimulation: Comparison with reaction time to acoustic, visual, and somatosensory stimuli. *Brain* 115: 109–122.

Pascual-Leone, A., Dhuna, A. K., and Gates, J. R. (1991b). Study of the frontal speech area with rapid-rate transcranial magnetic stimulation (abstract). *Electroencephalography and Clinical Neurophysiology* 85: 25P.

Pascual-Leone, A., Gates, J. R., and Dhuna, A. (1991c). Induction of speech arrest and counting errors with rapid-rate transcranial magnetic stimulation [see comments]. *Neurology* 41: 697–702.

Pascual-Leone, A., Valls-Solé, J., Brasil-Neto, J., Wassermann, E., Cohen, L. G., and Hallett, M. (1991d). Effect of focal transcranial magnetic stimulation on simple reaction time to visual, acoustic, and somatosensory stimuli. *Brain* 115: 1045–1059.

Pascual-Leone, A., Cammarota, A., Wassermann, E. M., Brasil-Neto, J. P., Cohen, L. G., and Hallett, M. (1993a). Modulation of motor cortical outputs to the reading hand of Braille readers. *Annals of Neurology* 34: 33–37.

Pascual-Leone, A., Cohen, L. G., Dang, N., Brasil-Neto, J. P., Cammarota, A., and Hallett, M. (1993b). Acquisition of new fine motor skills is associated with the modulation of cortical motor outputs (abstract). *Neurology* 43: A157.

Pascual-Leone, A., Houser, C. M., Reese, K., Shotland, L. I., Grafman, J., Sato, S., Valls-Solé, J., Brasil-Neto, J. P., Wassermann, E. M., Cohen, L., and Hallett, M. (1993c). Safety of rapid-rate transcranial magnetic stimulation in normal volunteers. *Electroencephalography and Clinical Neurophysiology* 89: 120–130.

Pascual-Leone, A., Grafman, J., and Hallett, M. (1994). Modulation of cortical motor output maps during development of implicit and explicit knowledge. *Science* 263: 1287–1289.

Pascual-Leone, A., Cohen, L. G., Brasil-Neto, J. P., Valls-Solé, J., and Hallett, M. (1994a). Differentiation of sensorimotor neuronal structures responsible for induction of motor evoked potentials, attenuation of detection of somatosensory stimuli, and induction of sensation of movement by mapping of optimal current directions. *Electroencephalography and Clinical Neurophysiology* 93: 230–236.

Pascual-Leone, A., Gomez-Tortosa, E., Grafman, J., Alway, D., Nichelli, P., and Hallett, M. (1994b). Induction of visual extinction by rapid-rate transcranial magnetic stimulation of parietal lobe [see comments]. *Neurology* 44 (pt. 1): 494–498.

Pascual-Leone, A., Valls-Solé, J., Wassermann, E. M., and Hallett, M. (1994c). Responses to rapid-rate transcranial magnetic stimulation of the human motor cortex. *Brain* 117 (pt. 4): 847–858.

Pascual-Leone, A., Nguyet, D., Cohen, L. G., Brasil-Neto, J. P., Cammarota, A., and Hallett, M. (1995a). Modulation of muscle responses evoked by transcranial magnetic stimulation during the acquisition of new fine motor skills. *Journal of Neurophysiology* 74: 1037–1045.

Pascual-Leone, A., Wassermann, E. M., Sadato, N., and Hallett, M. (1995b). The role of reading activity on the modulation of motor cortical outputs to the reading hand in Braille readers. *Annals of Neurology* 38: 910–915.

Pascual-Leone, A., Wassermann, E. M., Grafman, J., and Hallett, M. (1996). The role of the dorsolateral prefrontal cortex in implicit procedural learning. *Experimental Brain Research* 107: 479–485.

Pascual-Leone, A., Hamilton, R., Tormos, J. M., Keenan, J., and Catala, M. D. (1998a). Neuroplasticity in adjustment to blindness. In *Neuroplasticity: Building a Bridge from the Laboratory to the Clinic.* Berlin: Springer.

Pascual-Leone, A., Tormos, J. M., Keenan, J., Tarazona, F., Canete, C., and Catala, M. D. (1998b). Study and modulation of human cortical excitability with transcranial magnetic stimulation. *Journal of Clinical Neurophysiology* 15: 333–343.

Pascual-Leone, A., Bartres-Faz, D., and Keenan, J. P. (1999). Transcranial magnetic stimulation: Studying the brain-behaviour relationship by induction of "virtual lesions." *Philosophical Transactions of the Royal Society of London B, Biological Sciences* 354: 1229–1238.

Pascual-Leone, A., Tarazona, F., Keenan, J. P., Tormos, J. M., Hamilton, R., and Catala, M. D. (1999b). Transcranial magnetic stimulation and neuroplasticity. *Neuropsychologia* 37: 207–217.

Pascual-Leone, A., Walsh, V., and Rothwell, J. (2000). Transcranial magnetic stimulation in cognitive neuroscience: Virtual lesion, chronometry, and functional connectivity. *Current Opinion in Neurobiology* 10: 232–237.

Pascual-Leone, A., Davey, N., Wassermann, E. M., Rothwell, J., and Puri, B. K. (eds.). (2002). *Handbook of Transcranial Magnetic Stimulation.* London: Arnold.

Pascual-Leone, A., Cohen, L. G., Brasil-Neto, J. P., and Hallett, M. (1994). Noninvasive differention of motor cortical representation of hand muscles by mapping optimal current directions. *Electroencephalography and Clinical Neurophysiology* 93: 42–48.

Pashler, H. E. (1998). *The Psychology of Attention.* Cambridge, Mass.: MIT Press.

Paulus, W., Hallett, M., Rossini, P. M., and Rothwell, J. C. (1999). Transcranial magnetic stimulation. *Electroencephalography and Clinical Neurophysiology* supp 51.

Paus, T. (1999). Imaging the brain before, during, and after transcranial magnetic stimulation. *Neuropsychologia* 37: 219–224.

Paus, T., and Wolforth, M. (1998). Transcranial magnetic stimulation during PET: Reaching and verifying the target site. *Human Brain Mapping* 6: 399–402.

Paus, T., Jech, R., Thompson, C. J., Comeau, R., Peters, T., and Evans, A. C. (1997). Transcranial magnetic stimulation during positron emission tomography: A new method for studying connectivity of the human cerebral cortex. *Journal of Neuroscience* 17: 3178–3184.

Paus, T., Jech, R., Thompson, C. J., Comeau, R., Peters, T., and Evans, A. C. (1998). Dose-dependent reduction of cerebral blood flow during rapid-rate transcranial magnetic stimulation of the human sensorimotor cortex. *Journal of Neurophysiology* 79: 1102–1107.

Payne, B. R., and Lomber, S. G. (1999). A method to assess the functional impact of cerebral connections on target populations of neurons. *Journal of Neuroscience Methods* 86: 195–208.

Penfield, W., and Boldrey, E. (1937). Somatic motor and sensory representation in the cerebral cortex of man as studied by electrical stimulation. *Brain* 60: 389–443.

Penfield, W., and Jasper, H. (1954). *Epilepsy and the Functional Anatomy of the Human Brain.* Boston: Little and Brown.

Penfield, W., and Rasmussen, T. (1949). Vocalization and arrest of speech. *Archives of Neurological Psychiatry* 61: 21–27.

Penfield, W., and Rasmussen, T. (1950). *The Cerebral Cortex of Man.* 4th ed. New York: Macmillan.

Penfield, W., and Roberts, L. (1959). *Speech and Brain Mechanisms.* Princeton, N.J.: Princeton University Press.

Perry, R. J., and Zeki, S. (2000). The neurology of saccades and covert shifts in spatial attention: An event-related fMRI study. *Brain* 123: 2273–2288.

Peterhans, E., and von der Heydt, R. (1991). Subjective contours: Bridging the gap between psychophysics and physiology. *Trends in Neuroscience* 14: 112–119.

Piazza, M., Mechelli, A., Butterworth, B., and Price, C. J. (Submitted). Are subitizing and counting implemented as separate or functionally overlapping processes?

Poldrack, R. A. (2000). Imaging brain plasticity: Conceptual and methodological issues. A theoretical review. *NeuroImage* 12: 1–13.

Polson, M. J. R., Barker, A. T., and Freeston, I. L. (1982). Stimulation of nerve trunks with time-varying magnetic fields. *Medical and Biological Engineering and Computing* 20: 243–244.

Pons, T. P., Garraghty, P. E., Ommaya, A. K., Kaas, J. H., Taub, E., and Mishkin, M. (1991). Massive cortical reorganisation after sensory deafferentation in adult macaques. *Science* 252: 1857–1860.

Porter, R., and Lemon, R. (1993). *Corticospinal Function and Voluntary Movement.* Oxford: Oxford University Press.

Posner, M. I. (1978). *Chronometric Explorations of Mind.* Hillsdale, N.J.: Lawrence Erlbaum.

Posner, M. I., Walker, J. A., Friedrich, F. J., and Rafal, R. D. (1984). Effects of parietal lobe injury on covert orienting of visual attention. *Journal of Neuroscience* 4: 1863–1874.

Post, A., Muller, M. B., Engelmann, M., and Keck, M. E. (1999). Repetitive transcranial magnetic stimulation in rats: Evidence for a neuroprotective effect in vitro and in vivo. *European Journal of Neuroscience* 11: 3247–3254.

———

Presenti, M., Thioux, M., Seron, X., and De Volder, A. (2000). Neuroanatomical substrates of arabic number processing, numerical comparison, and simple addition: A PET study. *Journal of Cognitive Neuroscience* 12: 461–479.

Price, C. J., Wise, R. J. S., and Frackowiack, R. S. J. (1996). Demonstrating the implicit processing of visually presented words and pseudowords. *Cerebral Cortex* 6: 62–70.

Price, C. J., Mummery, C. J., Moore, C. J., Frackowiak, R. S. J., and Friston, K. J. (1999). Delineating necessary and sufficient neural systems with functional imaging studies of neuropsychological patients. *Journal of Cognitive Neuroscience* 11: 371–382.

Pridmore, S., and Belmaker, R. (1999). Transcranial magnetic stimulation in the treatment of psychiatric disorders. *Psychiatry and Clinical Neurosciences* 53: 541–548.

Priori, A., Bertolasi, L., Rothwell, J. C., Day, B. L., and Marsden, C. D. (1993). Some saccadic eye movements can be delayed by transcranial magnetic stimulation of the cerebral cortex in man. *Brain* 116 (pt. 2): 355–367.

Ramón y Cajal, S. (1894). La fine structure des centres nerveux. *Proceedings of the Royal Society of London* 55: 444–468.

Ramón y Cajal, S. (1904). Textura del sistema nervioso del hombe y de los vertibrados. Madrid: Nicolas Moya.

Ramón y Cajal, S. (1924). *Studies on Degeneration and Regeneration of the Nervous System*. Translated by R. M. May. London: Oxford University Press.

Ranck, J. B. (1975). Which elements are excited in electrical stimulation of the mammalian central nervous system? A review. *Brain Research* 98: 417–440.

Rauscheker, J. (1995). Compensatory plasticity and sensory substitution in the sensory cortex. *Trends in Neuroscience* 18: 36–43.

Reilly, J. P. (1992). *Electrical Stimulation and Electropathology.* Cambridge: Cambridge University Press.

———

Ridding, M. C., Sheean, G., Rothwell, J. C., Inzelberg, R., and Kujirai, T. (1995). Changes in the balance between motor cortical excitation and inhibition in focal, task specific dystonia. *Journal of Neurology, Neurosurgery, and Psychiatry* 59: 493–498.

Riopelle, A. J., and Ades, H. W. (1953). Visual discrimination performance in rhesus monkeys following extirpation of prestriate and temporal cortex. *Journal of General Psychology* 83: 63–77.

Riopelle, A. J., Alper, R. G., Strong, P. N., and Ades, H. W. (1953). Multiple discrimination and patterned string performance of normal and temporal lobectomied monkeys. *Journal of Comparative Physiology and Psychology* 46: 145–149.

Rizzolati, G., Fogassi, L., and Gallese, V. (1997). Parietal cortex: From sight to action. *Current Opinion in Neurobiology* 7: 562–567.

Ro, T., Cheifet, S., Ingle, H., Shoup, R., and Rafal, R. (1999). Localization of the human frontal eye fields and motor hand area with transcranial magnetic stimulation and magnetic resonance imaging. *Neuropsychologia* 37: 225–232.

Roberts, D. R., Vincent, D. J., Speer, A. M., Bohning, D. E., Cure, J., Young, J., and George, M. S. (1997). Multi-modality mapping of motor cortex: Comparing echoplanar BOLD fMRI and transcranial magnetic stimulation. Short communication. *Journal of Neural Transmission* 104: 833–843.

Robertson, E., Tormos, J. M., Maeda, F., and Pascual-Leone, A. (2001). The role of the dorsolateral prefrontal cortex during sequence learning is specific for spatial information. *Cerebral Cortex* 11: 628–635.

Robertson, I. H., and Murre, J. M. J. (1999). Rehabilitation of brain damage: Brain plasticity and principles of guided recovery. *Psychological Bulletin* 125: 544–575.

Rossi, S., Pasqualetti, P., Rossini, P. M., Feige, B., Ulivelli, M., Glocker, F. X., Battistini, N., Lucking, C. H., and Kresteva-Friege, R. (2000). Effects of repetitive transcranial magnetic stimulation on movement-related cortical activity in humans. *Cerebral Cortex* 10: 802–808.

Rossini, P. M., and Pauri, F. (2000). Neuromagnetic integrated methods tracking brain mechanisms of sensorimotor areas "plastic" reorganisation. *Brain Research Reviews* 33: 131–154.

Rossini, P. M., and Rossi, S. (1998). Clinical applications of motor evoked potentials (editorial). *Electroencephalography and Clinical Neurophysiology* 106: 180–194.

Rostomily, R. C., Berger, M. S., Ojemann, G., and Lettich, E. (1991). Postoperative deficits and functional recovery following removal of tumours involving the dormant hemisphere. *Journal of Neurosurgery* 75: 62–68.

Roth, B. J., Saypol, J. M., Hallett, M., and Cohen, L. G. (1991). A theoretical calculation of the field induced in the cortex during magnetic stimulation. *Electroencephalography and Clinical Neurophysiology* 81: 47–56.

Roth, B. J., Pascual-Leone, A., Cohen, L. G., and Hallett, M. (1992). The heating of metal electrodes during rapid rate magnetic stimulation: A possible safety hazard. *Electroencephalography and Clinical Neurophysiology* 85: 116–123.

Rothwell, J. C. (1993). Evoked potentials, magnetic stimulation studies, and event-related potentials. *Current Opinion in Neurology* 6: 715–723.

Rothwell, J. C. (1994). Motor cortical stimulation in man. In *Biomagnetic Stimulation,* S. Ueno (ed.). New York: Plenum Press, pp. 49–58.

Rothwell, J. C. (1997). Techniques and mechanisms of action of transcranial stimulation of the human motor cortex. *Journal of Neuroscience Methods* 74: 113–122.

Rugg, M. D., and Allen, K. (2000). Memory retrieval: An electrophysiological perspective. In *The New Cognitive Neurosciences,* M. S. Gazzaniga (ed.). Cambridge, Mass.: MIT Press, pp. 805–816.

Ruohonen, J., Ravazzani, P., Ilmoniemi, R. J., Galardi, G., Nilsson, J., Panizza, M., Amadio, S., Grandori, F., and Comi, G. (1996). Motor cortex mapping with combined MEG and magnetic stimulation. *Electroencephalography and Clinical Neurophysiology* supp. 46: 317–322.

Ruohonen, J., and Ilmoniemi, R. J. (1999). Modelling of the stimulating field generation in TMS. *Electroencephalography and Clinical Neurophysiology* supp. 51: 30–40.

Rumelhart, D. E., McClelland, J. L., and The PDP Research Group (1986). *Parallel Distributed Processing: Explorations in the Microstructure of Cognition.* Cambridge, Mass.: The MIT Press.

Rushworth, M. F., and Walsh, V. (eds.). (1999). *Transcranial Magnetic Stimulation in Neuropsychology. Neuropsychologia* 37 (special issue).

Rushworth, M. F., Nixon, P. D., Wade, D. T., Renowden, S., and Passingham, R. E. (1998). The left hemisphere and the selection of learned actions. *Neuropsychologia* 36: 11–24.

Rushworth, M. F. S., Ellison, A., and Walsh, V. (2001). Complementary localization of visual attention and motor intention. *Nature Neuroscience* 4: 656–661.

Sadato, N., Pascual-Leone, A., Grafman, J., Ibanez, V., Deiber, M. P., Dold, G., and Hallett, M. (1996). Activation of primary visual cortex by Braille reading in blind subjects. *Nature* 380: 526–528.

Salmelin, R., Hari, R., Lounasmaa, O. V., and Sams, M. (1994). Dynamics of brain activation during picture naming. *Nature* 368: 463–465.

Sathian, K., Simon, T. J., Peterson, S., Patel, G. A., Hoffman, J. L., and Grafton, S. T. (1999). Neural evidence linking visual object enumeration and attention. *Journal of Cognitive Neuroscience* 11: 36–51.

Sawaki, L., Okita, T., Fukiwara, M., and Mizumo, K. (1999). Specific and non-specific effects of transcranial magnetic stimulation upon simple and go/no-go reaction time. *Experimental Brain Research* 127: 402–408.

Schiller, F. (1953). Franz Gall. In *The Founders of Neurology,* W. Haymaker and F. Schiller (eds.). Springfield, Ill.: C. C. Thomas, pp. 31–35.

Schluter, N. D., Rushworth, M. F., Mills, K. R., and Passingham, R. E. (1999). Signal-, set-, and movement-related activity in the human premotor cortex. *Neuropsychologia* 37: 233–243.

Schluter, N. D., Rushworth, M. F., Passingham, R. E., and Mills, K. R. (1998). Temporary interference in human lateral premotor cortex suggests dominance for the selection of movements: A study using transcranial magnetic stimulation. *Brain* 121 (pt. 5): 785–799.

Schmolesky, M. T., Wang, Y., Hanes, D. P., Thompson, K. G., Leutgeb, S., Schall, J. D., and Leventhal, A. G. (1998). Signal timing across the macaque visual system 79: 3272–3278.

Schoppig, A., Clarke, S., Walsh, V., Assal, G., Meuli, R., and Cowey, A. (1999). Short-term memory for colour following posterior hemispheric lesions in man. *Neuroreport* 10: 1379–1384.

Seidel, D. (1968). Der exustenzbereich Elektrisch und magnetischinduktiv angeregter subjecktiver Lichterscheinungen (Phosphene) in Abhangigkeit von ausseren Reizparametern. *Elektromedizin* 13: 194–206, 208–211.

Seyal, M., Ro, T., and Rafal, R. (1995). Increased sensitivity to ipsilateral cutaneous stimuli following transcranial magnetic stimulation of the parietal lobe. *Annals of Neurology* 38: 264–267.

Shallice, T. (1988). *The Neuropsychology of Mental Structure.* Cambridge: Cambridge University Press.

Shapiro, K. A., Pascual-Leone, A., Mottaghy, F. M., Gangitand, M., and Caramazza, A. (2001). Grammatical distinctions in the left-frontal cortex. *Journal of Cognitive Neuroscience* 13: 713–720.

Shepard, S., and Metzeler, D. (1971). Mental rotation of three dimensional objects. *Science* 171: 701–703.

Shulman, G. L., Ollinger, J. M., Akbudak, E., Conturo, T. E., Snyder, A. Z., Petersen, S. E., and Corbetta, M. (1999). Areas involved in encoding and applying directional expectations to moving objects. *Journal of Neuroscience* 19: 9480–9496.

Siebner, H. R., Willoch, F., Peller, M., Auer, C., Boecker, H., Conrad, B., and Bartenstein, P. (1998). Imaging brain activation induced by long trains of repetitive transcranial magnetic stimulation. *Neuroreport* 9: 943–948.

Simon, H. A. (1981). *The Sciences of the Artificial*. Cambridge, Mass.: MIT Press.

Singh, K. D., Hamdy, S., and Aziz, Q. (1997). Topographic mapping of transcranial magnetic stimulation data on surface rendered MR images of the brain. *Electroencephalography and Clinical Neurophysiology* 105: 345–351.

Snyder, L. H., Batista, A. P., and Andersen, R. A. (1997). Coding of intention in the posterior parietal cortex. *Nature* 386: 167–169.

Sparing, R., Mottaghy, F. M., Ganis, G., Thompson, W. T., Töpper, R., Kosslyn, S. M., and Pascual-Leone, A. (2002). Visual cortex excitability increases during visual mental imagery: A TMS study in healthy human subjects. *Brain Research* 938: 92–97.

Sprague, J. M. (1966). Interaction of cortex and superior colliculus in mediation of visually guided behaviour in the cat. *Science* 154: 1544–1547.

Stadler, M. A. (1994). Explicit and implicit learning and maps of cortical motor output (letter, comment). *Science* 265: 1600–1601.

Stanescu-Cosson, R., Pinel, P., van de Moortele, P.-F., Le Bihan, D., Cohen, L., and Dehaene, S. (2000). Understanding dissociations in dyscalculia: A brain imaging study of the impact of number size on the cerebral networks for exact and approximate calculation. *Brain* 123: 2240–2255.

Stefan, K., Kunesch, E., Cohen, L. G., Benecke, R., and Classen, J. (2000). Induction of plasticity in the human motor cortex by paired pulse stimulation. *Brain* 123: 572–584.

Stewart, L. M., Battelli, L., Walsh, V., and Cowey, A. (1999). Motion perception and perceptual learning studied by magnetic stimulation. *Electroencephalography and Clinical Neurophysiology* 51: 334–350.

Stewart, L. M., Frith, U., Meyer, B.-U., and Rothwell, J. (2000). TMS over BA37 impairs picture naming. *Neuropsychologia* 39: 1–6.

Stewart, L. M., Walsh, V., Frith, U., and Rothwell, J. C. (2001a). TMS produces two dissociable types of speech arrest. *NeuroImage* 13: 472–478.

———

Stewart, L. M., Walsh, V., and Rothwell, J. C. (2001). Motor and phosphene thresholds: A TMS correlation study. *Neuropsychologia* 39: 114–119.

Strafella, A. P., and Paus, T. (2000). Modulation of cortical excitability during action observation: A transcranial magnetic stimulation study. *Neuroreport* 11: 2289–2292.

Tanner, J. M., Whitehouse, R. H., and Takaishi, M. (1966). Standards from birth to maturity for height, weight, height velocity, and weight velocity: British children. *Archives of Disease of Childhood* 41: 454–613.

Tarazona, F., Tormos, J. M., Cañete, C., Catala, M. D., and Pascual-Leone, A. (1997). Modulation of motor cortical excitability by repetitive transcranial magnetic stimulation influences implicit learning. *Society for Neuroscience Abstracts* 23: 1964.

Terao, Y., Fukuda, H., Ugawa, Y., Hikosaka, O., Hanajima, R., Ferubayashi, T., Sakai, K., Miyauchi, S., Sasaki, Y., and Kanazawa, I. (1998a). Visualization of the information flow though the human oculomotor cortical regions by transcranial magnetic stimulation. *Journal of Neurophysiology* 80: 936–946.

Terao, Y., Ugawa, Y., Sakai, K., Miyauchi, S., Fukuda, H., Sasaki, Y., Takino, R., Hanajima, R., Ferubayashi, T., and Kanazawa, I. (1998b). Localising the site of magnetic brain stimulation by functional MRI. *Experimental Brain Research* 121: 145–152.

Tergau, F., Tormos, J. M., Paulus, W., Ziemann, U., and Pascual-Leone, A. (1997). Effects of repetitive transcranial magnetic stimulation on cortico-spinal and cortico-cortical excitability. *Neurology* 48: A107.

Theoret, H., Haque, J., and Pascual-Leone, A. (2001). Increased variability of paced finger tapping accuracy following repetitive magnetic stimulation of the cerebellum in humans. *Neuroscience Letters* 306: 29–32.

Thompson, S. P. (1910). A physiological effect of an alternating magnetic field. *Proceedings of the Royal Society of London (Biological Sciences).* B82: 396–399.

Topper, R., Mottaghy, F. M., Brugmann, M., Noth, J., and Huber, W. (1998). Facilitation of picture naming by focal transcranial magnetic stimulation of Wernicke's area. *Experimental Brain Research* 121: 371–378.

Treisman, A. (1988). Features and objects: The fourteenth Bartlett memorial lecture. *Quarterly Journal of Experimental Psychology* A40: 201–237.

Treisman, A. (1996). The binding problem. *Current Opinion in Neurobiology* 6: 171–178.

Triggs, W. J., Calvanio, R., and Levine, M. (1997). Transcranial magnetic stimulation reveals a hemispheric asymmetry correlate of intermanual differences in motor performance. *Neuropsychologia* 35: 1355–1363.

Trompetto, C., Assini, A., Buccolieri, A., Marchese, R., and Abbruzzese, G. (2000). Motor recovery following stroke: A transcranial magnetic stimulation study. *Clinical Neurophysiology* 111: 1860–1867.

Tulving, E., and Schacter, D. L. (1990). Priming and human memory systems. *Science* 247: 301–306.

Ueno, S. (ed.). (1994). *Biomagnetic Stimulation*. New York: Plenum Press.

Ueno, S., Tashiro, T., and Harada, K. (1988). Localized stimulation of neural tissues in the brain by means of a paired configuration of time-varying magnetic fields. *Journal of Applied Physics* 64: 5862–5864.

Ugawa, Y., Rothwell, J. C., Day, B. L., Thompson, P. D., and Marsden, C. D. (1991). Percutaneous electrical stimulation of corticospinal pathways at the level of the pyramidal decussation in humans. *Annals of Neurology* 29: 418–427.

Uhl, F., Franzen, P., Lindinger, G., Lang, W., and Deeke, L. (1991). On the functionality of the visually deprived occipital cortex in early blind persons. *Neuroscience Letters* 124: 256–259.

Valentinuzzi, M. (1962). Theory of magnetophosphenes. *American Journal of Medical Electronics* 1: 112–121.

Vallar, G. (1998). Spatial hemineglect in humans. *Trends in Cognitive Science* 2: 87–97.

Van der Kamp, W., Maassen VanDenBrink, A., Ferrari, M. D., and van Dijk, J. G. (1996). Inter-ictal cortical hyperexcitability in migraine patients demonstrated with transcranial magnetic stimulation. *Journal of the Neurological Sciences* 139: 106–110.

Valls-Solé, J., Pascual-Leone, A., Wassermann, E. M., and Hallett, M. (1992). Human motor evoked responses to paired transcranial magnetic stimuli. *Electroencephalography Clinical Neuro-physiology* 85: 355–364.

Vogels, R., and Orban, G. A. (1990). How well do response changes of striate neurons signal differences in orientation: A study in the discriminating monkey. *Journal of Neuroscience* 10: 3543–3558.

Wada, S., Kuboyta, H., Maita, S., Yamamoto, I., Yamaguchi, M., Andoh, T., Kawakami, T., Okumura, F., and Takenaka, T. (1996). Effects of stimulus waveform on magnetic nerve stimu-lation. *Japanese Journal of Applied Physiology* 35: 1983–1988.

Waldvogel, D., van Gelderen, P., Muellbacher, W., Ziemann, U., Immisch, I., and Hallett, M. (2000). The relative metabolic demand of inhibition and excitation. *Nature* 406: 995–998.

Walsh, P. (1946). Magnetic stimulation of the human retina. *Federal Proceedings* 5: 109–110.

Walsh, V. (1998). Brain mapping: Faradization of the mind. *Current Biology* 8: R8–R11.

Walsh, V. (2000). Reverse engineering the human brain. *Philosophical Transactions of the Royal Society of London A* 358: 497–511.

Walsh, V., and Butler, S. R. (1996). Different ways of looking at seeing. *Behavioural Brain Research* 76: 1-2, 1-3.

Walsh, V., and Cowey, A. (1998). Magnetic stimulation studies of visual cognition. *Trends in Cognitive Science* 2: 103–110.

Walsh, V., and Cowey, A. (2000). Transcranial magnetic stimulation and cognitive neuroscience. *Nature Reviews* 1: 73–79.

Walsh, V., and Rushworth, M. (1999). A primer of magnetic stimulation as a tool for neuropsychology. *Neuropsychologia* 37: 125–135.

Walsh, V., Ashbridge, E., and Cowey, A. (1998a). Cortical plasticity in perceptual learning demonstrated by transcranial magnetic stimulation. *Neuropsychologia* 36: 363–367.

Walsh, V., Ellison, A., Battelli, L., and Cowey, A. (1998b). Task-specific impairments and enhancements induced by magnetic stimulation of human visual area V5. *Proceedings of the Royal Society of London B (Biological Sciences)* 265: 537–543.

Walsh, V., Ellison, A., Ashbridge, E., and Cowey, A. (1999). The role of the parietal cortex in visual attention—hemispheric asymmetries and the effects of learning: A magnetic stimulation study. *Neuropsychologia* 37: 245–251.

Walsh, V., Le Mare, C., Blaimire, A., and Cowey, A. (2000). Normal discrimination performance accompanied by priming deficits in monkeys with V4 or TEO lesions. *Neuroreport* 11: 1459–1462.

Wanet-Defalque, M. C., Veraart, C., De Volder, A., Metz, R., Michel, C., Dooms, G., and Goffinet, A. (1988). High metabolic activity in the visual cortex of early blind human subjects. *Brain Research* 446: 369–373.

Wang, H., Wang, X., and Scheich, H. (1996). LTD and LTP induced by transcranial magnetic stimulation in auditory cortex. *Neuroreport* 7: 521–525.

Wang, H., Wang, X., Wetzel, W., and Scheich, H. (1999). Rapid rate transcranial magnetic stimulation in auditory cortex induces LTP and LTD and impairs discrimination learning of frequency modulated tones. *Electroencephalography and Clinical Neurophysiology* supp. 21: 361–368.

Warrington, E. K. (1982). The fractionation of arithmetical skills: A single case study. *Quarterly Journal of Experimental Psychology* 34A: 31–35.

Warrington, E. K., and James, M. (1967). Tachistoscopic number estimation in patients with unilateral lesions. *Journal of Neurology, Neurosurgery, and Psychiatry* 30: 468–474.

Wassermann, E. M. (1998). Risk and safety of repetitive transcranial magnetic stimulation: Report and suggested guidelines from the International Workshop on the Safety of Repetitive Transcranial Magnetic Stimulation, June 5–7, 1996. *Electroencephalography and Clinical Neurophysiology* 108: 1–16.

Wassermann, E. M., McShane, L. M., Hallett, M., and Cohen, L. G. (1992). Noninvasive mapping of muscle representations in human motor cortex. *Electroencephalography and Clinical Neurophysiology* 85: 1–8.

Wassermann, E. M., Pascual-Leone, A., and Hallett, M. (1994). Cortical motor representation of the ipsilateral hand and arm. *Experimental Brain Research* 100: 121–132.

Wassermann, E. M., Wang, B., Zeffiro, T. A., Sadato, N., Pascual-Leone, A., Toro, C., and Hallett, M. (1996). Locating the motor cortex on the MRI with transcranial magnetic stimulation and PET. *NeuroImage* 3: 1–9.

Watson, J. D. G., Myers, R., Frackowiak, R. S. J., Hajnal, J. V., Woods, R. P., Mazziotta, J. C., Shipp, S., and Zeki, S. (1993). Area V5 of the human brain: Evidence from a combined study using positron emission tomography and magnetic resonance imaging. *Cerebral Cortex* 3: 79–94.

Weintraub, S., and Mesulam, M. M. (1987). Right cerebral dominance in spatial attention: Further evidence based on ipsilateral neglect. *Archives in Neurology* 44: 621–625.

Weissman, J. D., Epstein, C. M., and Davey, K. R. (1992). Magnetic brain stimulation and brain size: Relevance to animal studies. *Electroencephalography and Clinical Neurophysiology* 85: 215–219.

Wilding, E. L., and Rugg, M. D. (1996). An event-related potential study of recognition memory with and without retrieval of source. *Brain* 119: 889–905.

Wilson, C. L., Babb, T. L., Halgren, E., and Crandall, P. H. (1983). Visual receptive fields and response properties of neurons in human temporal lobe and visual pathways. *Brain* 106: 473–502.

Wolfe, J. M. (1994). Visual search in continuous, naturalistic stimuli. *Vision Research* 34: 1187–1195.

Wolford, G., Miller, M. B., and Gazzaniga, M. (2000). The left hemisphere's role in hypothesis formation. *Journal of Neuroscience* 20: 1–4.

Young, M. P., Hilgetag, C., and Scannell, J. W. (1999). Models of paradoxical lesion effects and rules of inference for imputing function to structure in the brain. *Neurocomputing* 26–27: 933–938.

Young, M. P., Hilgetag, C., and Scannell, J. W. (2000). On imputing function to structure from the behavioural effects of brain lesions. *Proceeding of the Royal Society of London* 355: 147–161.

Zanette, G., Tinazzi, M., Bonato, C., di Summa, A., Manganoti, P., Polo, A., and Fiaschi, A. (1997). Reversible changes of motor cortical outputs following immobilization of the upper limb. *Electroencephalography and Clinical Electrophysiology* 105: 269–279.

Zangaladze, A., Epstein, C. M., Grafton, S. T., and Sathian, K. (1999). Involvement of visual cortex in tactile discrimination of orientation. *Nature* 401: 587–590.

Zangemeister, W. H., Canavan, A. G., and Hoemberg, V. (1995). Frontal and parietal transcranial magnetic stimulation (TMS) disturbs programming of saccadic eye movements. *Journal of the Neurological Sciences* 133: 1–2, 42–52.

Zatorre, R., Perry, D. W., and Beckett, C. A. (1998). Functional anatomy of musical processing in listeners with absolute pitch. *Proceedings of the National Academy of Sciences, U.S.A.* 95: 3172–3177.

Zeki, S. (1993). *A Vision of the Brain.* London: Blackwell Scientific.

Ziemann, U., and Hallett, M. (2000). Basic neurophysiological studies with TMS. In *Transcranial Magnetic Stimulation in Neuropsychiatry,* M. A. George and M. Bellmaker (eds.). Washington, D. C.: American Psychiatric Press, pp. 45–98.

Ziemann, U., Rothwell, J. C., and Ridding, M. C. (1996). Interaction between intracortical inhibition and facilitation in human motor cortex. *Journal of Physiology* 496: 873–881.

Ziemann, U., Steinhoff, B. J., Tergau, F., and Paulus, W. (1998). Transcranial magnetic stimulation: Its current role in epilepsy research. *Epilepsy Research* 30: 11–30.

Zihl, J., von Cramon, D. O., and Mai, N. (1983). Selective disturbance of movement vision after bilateral brain damage. *Brain* 106: 313–340.

Name Index

Abdeen, M. A., 44

Ades, H. W., 3

Afra, J., xvii, 204

Aldini, G., 21, 23

Allen, K., 2, 223

Amassian, V. E., 44, 46, 50, 97, 99, 114, 125, 229

Anand, S., 73, 75

Andersen, R. A., 2, 133

Anderson, S. J., 2

Archibald, Y., 109

Arguin, M., 100

Artner, C., 204

Ashbridge, E., 50, 69, 76, 77, 79, 81–83, 100, 102, 127, 141, 142, 186, 187, 223

Ashby, P., 216

Aurora, S. K., xvii, 204

Bar, M., 148, 220

Barbur, J., 2, 125

Barker, A. T., 14, 16, 36–40, 42–44, 47, 49, 57

Barlow, H. B., 34–35

Bartolomeo, P., 209, 210

Bartres-Faz, D., 71, 73, 158

Baseler, H., 2

Batista, A. P., 133

Bavelier, D., 223

Bayer, R., 138

Beckers, G., 73, 76

Beer, B., 27, 30

Bellmaker, R. H., xvi, 217, 228

Berardelli, A., 78, 195

Bichot, N. P., 126

Bickford, R. G., 36

Biederman, I., 148, 220

Bisiach, E., 100, 129, 211

Bisley, J. W., 148, 192, 220

Bogdahn, U., 62

Bohning, D. E., 54, 219, 221

Bois-Reymond, E. D., 19

Boldrey, E., 27

Boroojerdi, B., 73, 75

Boulliaud, J. B., 199–200

Bowers, D., 129

Brasil-Neto, J. P., 46, 50, 169–171

Bravo, M. J., 190

Broca, P. P., 199, 200

Buckner, R. L., 2

Bullier, J., 123

Burnstine, T. H., 158

Bütefisch, C. M., 170, 223, 226, 227

Butler, S. R., 3

Butter, C. M., 3

Butterworth, B., 138

Cajal. *see* Ramón y Cajal, S.

Caldini, L., 19, 24

Campana, G., 76, 90, 148, 150, 192, 197, 220, 223

Canavan, A. G., 107, 109

Caramia, M. D., 204

Carlesimo, G. A., 147

Catano, A., 204

Cavada, C., 133

Cavanagh, P., 100

Celebrini, S., 99

Charcot, J.-M., 26

Chen, R., 78, 90, 91, 131, 155, 204, 216

Chez, G., 9

Chiappa, K. H., 51

Childer, J. G., 23–24

Chochon, F., 138

Chomsky, N., xiii

Chronicle, E. P., xvii

Classen, J., 170, 184, 186, 187, 197, 223, 226, 227

Claus, D., 80

Cloquet, J., 16

Cohen, J. D., 114

Coles, M. G. H., 4

Collin, N. G., 111

Corbetta, M., 2, 103

Corthout, E., 69, 77, 98, 149

Coslett, H. B., 210

Cowell, S. F., 3, 138

Cowey, A., 3, 4, 6, 7, 41, 50, 58, 60, 76–77, 79, 81–83, 90, 100, 102, 120, 127, 141, 142, 147, 148, 150, 186, 187, 192, 197, 220, 223, 229

Crick, F., 164

Critchley, M., 3

Damasio, A. R., 165, 205–206

Damasio, H., 3, 203, 205–206

D'Arsonval, A., 28, 29, 32

Davey, K. R., 229

Davey, N. J., 53

Davy, H., 17

Day, B. L., 50, 65–68, 78, 79, 97n, 106

Dehaene, S., 138

Delgado, J. M. R., 16

Demmer, I., 50

de Quervain, D., 79

Desimone, R., 153

Desmurget, M., 111

Donders, F. C., 3

Dorf, R. C., 166

Duchenne de Boulogne, G-B. Guillaume, 19–20, 22
Duncan, J., 96, 153
Dunlap, K., 32–33
Durand, D. M., 43

Edgeley, S. A., 229
Ellison, A., 82, 95, 103, 106, 109, 133–134, 143, 197
Epstein, C. M., 50, 157, 158, 229
Eyre, J. A., 166, 167, 169

Fadiga, L., 117
Faraday, M., 14, 16–18, 21–24
Farah, M., 148
Ferrier, D., 25–26, 200
Fierro, B., 50, 128–130, 211
Flament, D., 167, 170, 229
Flitman, S. S., 86, 157
Flourens, P., 24
Fogassi, L., 133
Fontana, F. G., 19, 21, 24
Foster, M. A., 40
Fox, P., 91, 219, 221
Frackowiak, R. S. J., 2, 158
Francois-Franck, C., 27
Freeston, I. L., 36, 44
Fremming, B. D., 36
Friedman-Hill, S. R., 100, 106
Fritsch, G., 25
Fuglsang-Frederiksen, A., 91

Gabrieli, J. D. E., 147
Gage, P., 202–203

Gallese, V., 133
Galvani, L., 17, 19
Ganis, G., 69, 77, 78, 116, 118
Garnham, C. W., 44
Gauld, A., 15
Gazzaniga, M., 147, 164
Geddes, L. A., 27, 33, 36
George, M. S., xvi, 54, 61, 217, 221
George, P., 9, 220
Gerloff, C., 111
Gibson, J. R., 77
Gilbert, W., 15
Gmelin, E., 16
Göbel, S., 138–140
Goldman-Rakic, P. S., 133
Golgi, C., 11–13
Goodale, M. A., 116
Grabowska, T. J., 165
Grafman, J., 159, 184, 186, 193
Granger, 19
Greenlee, M. W., 147, 149
Grosof, D. H., 220
Gross, C. G., 3

Hadjikhani, N., 2
Haenny, P. E., 116, 177
Haggard, P., 2–4, 83, 119, 120, 125
Hall, E. J., 170, 172, 229
Hall, S. T., 16
Hallett, M., 77, 80, 184, 186, 193, 195, 204
Haque, J., 216
Harada, K., 46
Harding, G. F. A., 2
Harlow, J., 202

Hausmann, A., 228

Hawken, M. J., 220

Heilman, K. M., 129

Heinen, F., 51, 55, 169

Hess, C. W., 51, 79, 82

Hilgetag, C. C., 152, 155, 156, 214

Hill, A. C., 53

Hillyard, S. A., 2, 223

Hinde, R. A., 167

Hitzig, E., 25

Hodgkin, A. L., 12

Holliday, I. E., 2

Hopkins, D. A., 167

Horel, J. A., 9, 220

Horsley, V., 27

Hotson, J. R., 73, 75–76, 120

Houa, M., 204

Hubel, D. H., 82–83

Hümberg, V., 107, 109

Humphreys, G. W., 96

Hupe, J. M., 9, 99

Huxley, A. F., 12

Ilmoniemi, R. J., 43, 55, 56, 62, 76, 115, 223

Inghilleri, 226

Ingvar, D., 158

Iwai, E., 3

Jackson, H., 24, 26

Jalinous, R., 40

James, F. A., 22, 24

James, M., 138

Jasper, H., 27, 201

Jennum, P., 90, 157

Jewell, G., 129

Jing, H., 224, 225

Joanette, Y., 100

Johansson, R. S., 7, 112, 113, 195

Kammer, T., 45, 50, 53, 72, 149

Kandel, E. R., 202

Kapur, N., 152, 152n, 214

Kastner, S., 50

Kawamichi, H., 117

Keck, M. E., 228

Keenan, J. P., 71, 73

Kelvin, Lord, 23

Kennard, C., 53

Kew, J. J., 169, 172, 173, 195

Kimura, D., 109

King, J. W., 223

Kinsbourne, M., 211

Koch, C., 164

Kolin, A., 35

Konogaya, M., 204

Konogaya, Y., 204

Kosslyn, S. M., 2, 7, 78, 92, 116, 131, 132, 220, 221

Kotter, R., 152

Krings, T., 77

Kuhn, T., 14

Kujirai, T., 80, 212

Kutas, M., 223

Kuypers, H. G. J. M., 167

Lawrence, D. G., 167

Lemon, R., 78

Lemon, R. J., 170

Lemon, R. N., 7, 112, 113, 195, 229

Le Roy, C., 19, 20

Lesser, 202

Libet, B., 119

Liepert, J., 75, 226

Lindsay, Lord, 23

Livingstone, M. S., 83

Lomber, S. G., 9, 140, 155, 206, 211

Lovsund, P., 35

Luck, S. J., 2, 223

Lueck, C. J., 2

Lynch, A. C., 32

Maccabee, P. J., 44

Maeda, F., 78, 91, 155, 204

Magno, E., 83, 119, 120, 125

Magnus, R., 14–15, 27

Magnussen, S., 147, 149

Magnusson, C. E., 33, 34

Malin, J.-P., 75

Maljkovic, V., 197, 220

Malpeli, J. G., 9

Mamoli, B., 204

Mangun, G. R., 2

Manning, F. J., 3

Mano, Y., 204

Mantel, G. W. H., 229

Marangolo, P., 148

Marg, E., xvii, 15, 29, 31, 34, 50

Marr, D., x, 3

Martin, J. H., 9

Martin-Elkins, C. L., 9, 220

Marzi, C. A., 86–88, 99, 116

Mateer, C., 158

Mathis, J., 79

Matteucci, C., 19

Maunsell, J. H. R., 77, 116, 177

McBride, E. R., 189

McClelland, J. L., x

McCourt, M. E., 129

McHenry, I. C., 199

McLeod, P., 153

McRobbie, D., 40

Meienberg, O., 82

Mendoza, D. W., 189

Merton, P. A., 37–38

Mesmer, F. A., 15, 16

Mesulam, M. M., 100, 140

Metzeler, D., 96

Meyer, B.-U., 46, 50

Meyer, D. E., 4

Michaels, C. F., 97

Miller, J. O., 4, 126

Miller, M. B., 147, 149, 164, 169

Miller, S., 166, 167

Mills, K. R., xvi, 4, 51, 80, 205

Milner, A. D., 116, 202

Milner, B., 3

Mishkin, M., 3

Monsul, N., 210

Moore, C. J., 158

Moran, J., 153

Morioka, T., 50

Morland, A. B., 2

Morton, H. B., 38

Mottaghy, F. M., 8, 207, 209, 216, 221

Moutoussis, K., 125

Moyer, R., 138

Muellbacher, W., 204

Muir, R. B., 229

Mulleners, W., xvii

Mulleners, W. M., 204

Müller, E. K., 28

Muller, M. B., 228

Münte, T. F., 223

Muri, R. M., 82, 108, 109

Murray, N. M. F., 38, 51

Murre, J. M. J., 153, 205

Nagarajan, S. S., 43

Nakayama, K., 190, 197, 220

Neville, H., 223

Niehaus, L., 62, 63

Noel, P., 204

Nowak, L. G., 77

Nusseck, H. G., 45

O'Breathnach, U., 79

Ohtsuka, K., 107

Ojemann, G., 158

Oliveri, M., xvi, 80, 115, 155, 211–215

Orban, G. A., 77

Oster, G., 35

Oyachi, H., 107

Paracelus, T., 15

Pardo, J., 140

Pascual-Leone, A., xvi, 4, 7, 50, 60–62, 70, 71, 73, 77–79, 82, 84, 90–91, 94, 99, 116, 120, 128, 129, 131, 147, 148, 155, 157, 169, 172, 175–179, 181, 182, 184–186, 188–191, 193–195, 204, 205, 216, 217, 223

Pashler, H. E., 4, 68

Pasternak, T., 148, 192, 220

Paulus, W., xvi, 4, 217

Pauri, F., 153

Paus, T., 51, 52, 117, 133, 219, 221

Pavlov, I., 27

Payne, B. R., 9, 155, 211

Penfield, W., 27, 81n, 158, 197, 201

Perry, R. J., 2

Peterhans, E., 220

Piazza, M., 138

Poldrack, R. A., 165

Polson, M. J. R., 36

Pons, T. P., 177

Porter, R., 78

Posner, M. I., 3, 96, 135

Post, A., 228

Presenti, M., 138

Price, C. J., 2, 158

Pridmore, S., 228

Priori, A., 79, 106–107

Quirk, G. J., 229

Rafal, R., 86, 88, 114, 153

Ramesh, V., 166, 167, 169

Ramón y Cajal, S., 12, 13, 166

Ranck, J. B., 55

Rasmussen, T., 27, 81n, 197

Rauscheker, J., 177

Reilly, J. P., 40, 44

Ridding, M. C., 204, 212, 226

Riopelle, A. J., 3

Rizzolati, G., 133

Ro, T., 82, 86, 88, 114, 153

Roberts, D. R., 221

Roberts, L., 158

Robertson, E., 216

Robertson, I. H., 153, 205

Robertson, L. C., 100, 106

Rolando, L., 24

Rosler, K. M., 82

Rossi, S., 77, 78, 203

Rossini, P. M., 77, 153, 204

Rostomily, R. C., 158

Roth, B. J., 40, 223

Rothstein, A. L., 189

Rothwell, J. C., 38, 51, 61, 73, 188, 195,
    212, 216, 226

Rowell, T. E., 167

Rudiak, D., xvii

Rugg, M. D., 2, 223

Rumelhart, D. E., x

Ruohonen, J., 43, 50

Rushworth, M. F. S., xvi, 2, 4, 71, 75, 82, 95,
    109, 119, 133–134, 138, 143, 148, 197

Sadato, N., 177

Salmelin, R., 2

Sathian, K., 138

Sawaki, L., 85–86

Scannell, J. W., 152

Schacter, D. L., 147

Schall, J. D., 126

Scheich, H., 90

Schiller, F., 116

Schiller, P. H., 177

Schluter, N. D., 2, 82, 83, 109, 112, 119

Schmolesky, M. T., 99

Schoppig, A., 3

Sechenov, I., 27

Seidel, D., 35

Seyal, M., 86, 88, 114, 115, 153

Shallice, T., 3, 4, 95

Shapiro, K. A., 160–162

Shapley, R. M., 220

Shepard, S., 96

Sherrington, C. S., 27

Siebner, H. R., 53, 54

Simon, H. A., x

Singh, K. D., 50

Snyder, L. H., 133

Sparing, R., 189–190

Spencer-Booth, Y., 167

Sprague, J. M., 152

Squire, L. R., 202

Stadler, M. A., 184

Stallings, 221

Stanescu-Cosson, R., 138

Stefan, K., 169, 195

Stevens, H. C., 33, 34

Stewart, A., 229

Stewart, L. M., 50, 61, 72–74, 76, 84, 92,
    120, 127, 158, 187, 188, 193, 197, 223

Stoerig, P., 7, 229

Strafella, A. P., 117

Stuchley, M. A., 44

Takaishi, M., 166

Takigawa, M., 224

Tanner, J. M., 166

Tarazona, F., 147, 193

Tashiro, T., 46

Teder-Sälejärvi, W. A., 223

Teggenthoff, M., 75

Terao, Y., 50, 84, 108

Tergau, F., 91

Theoret, H., 155, 216

Thompson, S. P., 23, 28–29, 31, 32

Topham, W., 16

Topper, R., 159

Torres, F., 116, 169, 175, 178, 179, 223

Treisman, A., 96, 100, 106

Triggs, W. J., 79

Trompetto, C., 204

Tulving, E., 147

Turvey, M. T., 97

Ueno, S., 46

Ugawa, Y., 195

Uhl, F., 177

Valentinuzzi, M., 35

Vallar, G., 100, 129, 211

Valls-Sole, J., 80

van der Kamp, W., 204

Vogels, R., 77

Volta, A., 19

von der Heydt, R., 220

Wada, S., 40

Waldvogel, D., 222

Walsh, P., 33–35

Walsh, V., xvi, 3, 4, 6, 7, 41, 45, 50, 58, 60, 61,
    71, 73, 75–77, 79, 81–83, 88, 90, 94, 95,
    99, 100, 102, 109, 120, 126, 127,
    133–134, 138, 141–143, 146, 148, 150,
    153, 154, 186–188, 192, 197, 220, 223

Wandell, B., 2

Wanet-Defalque, M. C., 177

Wang, H., 90

Wang, X., 90

Ward, W. S., 16

Warman, E. N., 43

Warrington, E. K., 138

Wassermann, E. M., 50, 61, 62, 77,
    78, 221

Watson, J. D. G., 2, 58, 70

Weintraub, S., 100

Weissman, J. D., 229

Westling, G., 7, 112, 113, 195

Whitehouse, R. H., 166

Wichman, H., 189

Wiesel, T. N., 82

Wilding, E. L., 2

Wilson, C. L., 99

Winkel, H., 90

Wise, R. J. S., 2, 158

Wolfe, J. M., 96

Wolford, G., 147, 164

Wolforth, M., 219

Wombell, J., 16

Young, M. P., 152

Zanette, G., 75, 214

Zangaladze, A., 69, 77, 99, 107, 109, 116,
    133, 177

Zeki, S., 2, 3, 73, 76, 125

Ziemann, U., 50, 80, 205, 212, 226

Zihl, J., 153

Subject Index

Acoustic artifacts, 86

Action (selection), xvi, 1, 2, 188

Activating functions, Barker's, 43–44

Akineptosia, 71

Alternating vs. direct current, 33–36

Amnesia, 202

Amputees, 169, 176
  congenital, 172, 173
  traumatic, 172–174

Anesthesia, mesmeric, 16

"Animal electricity," 19

Animal magnetism, 15–16

Animals, TMS and other, 228–229

Antisaccade task, 108

Aphémie, 199

Attention and inattention, xvi, 1, 2,
  133–137, 211

Auditory thresholds, 59–60

Awareness, xvi, 1, 7, 117, 119–123,
  125, 153

BA37, 158, 159

Back projections, 8, 99, 123

Basal ganglia, 55–56, 216

Behavioral assay, 82

Biphasic pulse, 40

Biphasic waveform, 40

Blindness, 19, 20, 121, 165, 175–178,
  181, 183. *See also* Braille reading
  early-blind subjects, 181

Braille reading, 175–183

Brain imaging, 2–3, 130. *See also*
  specific techniques
  TMS and, 221–222

Brain maps. *See* Mapping of the mind

Broca's area, 82, 160, 162, 201

Callosal connections, 116

Causal connections, 7

Central motor-conduction time
  (CCT), 51

Cerebral hemispheres, abnormal interaction between, 114

Chronometric causality, 125, 126, 183

Cingulate cortex, 140

Cognitive contours, 220

Cognitive function, theories of grounding/evaluating, xiii

Cognitive neuroscience, development of, ix

Cognitive resolution, 1–10, 55

Coils, 17–24, 32–34, 44
  circular, 45–47, 49, 106
  figure-of-eight, 45–47, 49, 51, 57
  and neurons, 45–49

Color aftereffect, 73, 74

Color-discrimination task, 190, 192

Color perception, 2, 3, 125

Color priming, 151

Compensation, neural, 9, 140

Compensatory analysis, 205–207, 209, 214

Compensatory modulation, 214

Competition
  between areas within a hemisphere, 153
  between hemispheres, 153, 155, 211
    (see also Hemispheres)
  between stimuli, 153

Computer metaphor, ix–x

Conduction times, constant, 166

Consciousness. See Awareness

Consciousness studies, 1

Cooling, 9

Cortex, electric stimulation of, 24–28

Cortical excitability, 78, 155, 172, 188–190, 204, 214, 216–217. See also Epileptic seizures
  caused by TMS, 89–92
  low-frequency rTMS decreases, 90

Cortical interactions, 5, 80

Cortical reorganization, 89, 174–177.
    See also Plasticity; Reorganization

Current flow. See also Alternating vs. direct current
  how it activates neurons, 43

Depression (cortical), long-term, 90

Depression (mental illness), 17, 61

Descriptive adequacy, xiii

Developmental motor studies, 169

Dextromethorphan, 226

Direct current. See Alternating vs. direct current

Disruptive mode of TMS, 45, 83, 84, 89

Distal method, 90, 91, 155, 223, 229

Drugs, TMS and, 226–228

Dual-task experiments, 4, 62

Dyslexia, 210

Ear plugs, 60

Elaboration areas, 81, 197

Electric fields induced by TMS, 44, 46–48, 50
  as function of depth, 57

Electric stimulation of cortex, 24–28, 50–51

Electricity, internal. See Muscle current

Electroencephalogram (EEG), xv, 37, 55–56, 68
off-line, 223
TMS and, 222–225
Electromagnetic induction, discovery of, 14
Electromyogram (EMG), 51, 65–68, 112, 113
Epileptic seizures, 61, 201–202, 204–205
Event-related potentials (ERPs), 2, 3, 5, 6, 69, 77, 79, 223–225
Explanatory adequacy, xiii
Extinction, 50, 128, 129, 211–215
Eye, electromagnet applied to, 28
Eye movements, xvi, 2, 35, 95, 100, 106

Face twitches, 60
Facilitations, 84–88
intersensory, 84, 86
paradoxical functional, 152–156
Faradization, 20–24
Focality of TMS, 46, 49–56. *See also* Spatial resolution
Form-from-color processing, 76
Form-from-motion processing, 76
Frontal eye fields (FEFs), 52, 82, 108, 111, 133
Frontal lobe, 50, 52, 82, 108, 111,125, 133, 158, 199–202
Functional magnetic resonance imaging (fMRI), xi, xv, 2, 3, 5, 50, 51, 54, 221, 222

GABA (γ-aminobutyric acid), 226
Gerstmann's syndrome, 138

"Go/no go" task, 85–86
Grammar. *See under* Language

"Hand passing," 16–17
Healing through "magnetism," 15–16
Hemianopic subjects, 121, 123
Hemispheres, interaction between, 86–88, 115, 128, 153, 155, 211, 213
History, 11–38
of magnetic brain stimulation, 14
neuron(al) theory, 12
reticular nervous system, 12
H.M., 202
Homunculus, 27, 50
Hunting paradigm, 81, 82

Illusory contours, 220
Imagery
motor, 189
visual, 1, 92, 116, 117, 132, 190
Implicit learning, 165
Implicit motor learning, 147
Implicit motor-learning task, 193
Implicit-sequence learning task, 184
Information processing, 126, 192. *See also specific topics*
Intention, 95. *See also* Motor attention
Interhemispheric competition. *See* Hemispheres
Intracortical excitation, 226
Intracortical inhibition, 212

Language, 1, 2
nouns and verbs, xvi, 160–162

Language perception and production, 83–84, 201. *See also* Speech
   rTMS and, 160–162
Language processing, studies of, 157–159
Language-related memory function, 159
Latency. *See* Reaction time
Lesion analysis, 205–206
   logic of, 4, 8, 9
Lesion effects, paradoxical, 214
Lesions
   primary and secondary, 195
   reversibility, 8–9
Localization of function, 24–25, 200, 206
Lodestone, 15
Longitudinal studies, 167
Long term potentiation, 90, 193
Lorazepam, 226

Magnetic "cures," 15
Magnetic induction, Faraday's discovery of, 17–18, 22–24
Magnetic stimulators, circuitry of, 39
Magnetic substance, first discovery of, 14–15
Magnetism
   ancient roots, 14–17
   healing power, 15–16
   origin of term, 15
"Magnetite," 15
Magnetoencephalopathy (MEG), xv, 2, 3, 5–6, 50, 68, 69
Magnetophosphenes, 28–29, 31, 32, 35
Mapping the mind
   assumptions and expectations, 220–221
   multidimensional, 219–220

Masking paradigm, 4. *See also* Visual masking
Memory, xvi, 1, 2, 159, 202. *See also* Perceptual memory
   working, 149, 207, 209
Memory-guided saccades, 106–109
Mental imagery, 116–117, 131, 132, 189–190
Mental rotation, 77, 116–118
Mesmeric sleep, 16
Mesmerism, 15
Methodological considerations, 93.
   See also Facilitations; Repetitive-pulse methodology; Single-pulse methodology; Stimulation
   guidelines on experimental procedure, 70
   silent periods and paired-pulse paradigms, 79–80, 94
Migraineurs, xvii
Mind and brain, relation between, ix
Mirror movements, 204
Monkeys
   macque, 167
   TMS in, 228–229
Monophasic pulse, 40, 46
Motion aftereffect, 73, 74
"Motion blind" patient, 153
Motion coherence thresholds, 66
Motion deficits, 76
Motion-detection/discrimination task, 71, 193, 195–197
Motion discrimination, 76
Motion perception, 2, 3, 70, 71, 125. *See also* Awareness
Motion priming, 148, 150

Motor areas, differences between, 111–112

Motor attention, 136, 137. *See also* Intention

Motor cortex, 38, 53, 54, 109, 116, 117, 119, 156, 158, 159, 165, 184. *See also* Cortical excitability

 magnetic stimulation of, 38, 55–56, 109

 supplemental, 111

Motor-evoked potentials (MEPs), 75, 77, 79–81, 117, 169, 171, 184, 188, 195

Motor homunculus, 50

Motor neuron disease, 38

Motor selection, effects of TMS on, 109–111

Motor skill-learning tasks, 186–187, 191, 193

Motor thresholds, 61, 77–78, 167

Movement evoked by electric stimulation, 24–26

Movements, timing of, 166

Multiple sclerosis (MS), 38

Muscle current, 17, 19–20

N-methyl-D-aspartate (NMDA), 226

Naming, 158–159

Neglect, 50, 95, 211, 212, 214

 modeling, 128–130

Nerve stimulator, magnetic, 39, 40

Neural network models, x

Neural noise, 45, 62, 66, 68, 69, 93. *See also* Virtual lesions

Neurochronometry, 125–126

Neurons, stimulation of, 43–44

Neurophysiology, clinical, xvi

Neuropsychiatry, xvi

Neuropsychological studies, problems with, 95–96

Neuropsychology, limits of, 95–96

Number line, 138, 139

Number Stroop, 140

Numerical representation and manipulation, xvi, 138–140

Object naming, 158–159

Observational adequacy, xiii

Occipital cortex, see visual areas and visual cortex

"Off-line" paradigm. *See* Distal method

Operculum, left frontal, 199–200

Orientation columns in V1, 82–83

Orienting, 82, 114, 128–129, 133–137

Paired-pulse paradigms, 80, 94, 212, 214

Paresthesias, 114

Parietal cortex, 85, 100, 115, 125, 133, 148, 153, 156, 211, 228. *See also* Memory-guided saccades

 changing role in visual search, 186–187

 damage to, 95, 138, 211–213

 posterior parietal cortex (PPC), 82, 100, 105–109, 111, 133, 135, 139, 140, 142, 143, 148, 150, 173 (*see also under* Visual search tasks)

 right vs. left, 95, 105, 111, 128–130, 138, 140, 155

Perception, xvi, 1

Perceptual learning, 140–147

Perceptual memory, as new window for TMS and psychophysics, 147–151

Perceptual representation system (PRS), 147, 148. *See also* Perceptual memory
Phantom-limb phenomenon, 170–174
Phonological retrieval, 158–159
Phosphene thresholds, 73, 75, 121, 190, 193
  modulation, 190
  stability over time, 73
Phosphenes, xvi, 20, 28, 32, 33, 35, 50, 72, 78, 81, 121–124
  electrophosphenes, 19
  magnetophosphenes, 28–29, 31, 32, 35
  moving, 72, 73, 123, 193
  production of moving visual, 72–73, 193
Phrenology, 16
Phrenomagnetism, 16
Picture naming, 158–159
Plasticity, xvi, 80, 163–166, 172, 176, 183–188, 195, 197, 214, 226. *See also* Phantom limb phenomenon
  childhood development and, 166 170
  compensatory, 8
  in the context of normal behavior, 164–165
  guiding change, 192–196
  modulation, 195
  necessities following insufficiencies, 174–183
  on-line, 197
  over short time periods, 169
  real-time, 183
  specter of neural compensation, 9

Positron emission tomography (PET), xi, xv, 2, 3, 5, 50, 51, 54, 207
Practice, 170
  physical and mental, 188–192
  structured mental practice, 189
  plasticity with, 183–188
Prefrontal cortex, 61, 203, 207
  dorsolateral, 8, 193, 194, 207
Premotor cortex, 82, 109–111, 119, 121
Premotor processes, awareness of, 119
Priming, xvi, 147–151, 153, 192
  conceptual, 147
  perceptual, 147
"Problem space," 6
Procedural learning, 194
Processing systems, theories of, xi
Productive mode, 45
Pseudoneglect, 129, 211
"Psychocivilized society," 16
Psychological refractory period (PRP), 223–224
Pulse, monophasic and biphasic, 40, 46
Pulse strength and behavioral effects, 59, 60
Pulsed magnetic fields, and modern era of magnetic stimulation, 36–38

Rats, 228
Reach-lift task, 113
Reaction time (RT), 65, 66, 68, 85.
  See also Facilitations; Serial reaction-time test
  of voluntary movement, 78
Reading, 209–210

Regional cerebral blood flow (rCBF), 52, 53, 207, 209
safety, 59, 61–63
Rehearsal, mental, 188–189
Relative timing of processes, 100–109
Reorganization, 8, 128, 170, 177. *See also* Cortical reorganization
Repetitive-pulse methodology, 76, 81–83, 89, 90, 127–162
Repetitive pulse (rTMS), 5–6, 8, 39–41, 53, 58, 131, 148, 158–159, 209, 214, 216, 228
changes in sensitivity of cortex and, 78
distal, 90–93
excitability of motor cortex by, 91–92
and future of virtual patients, 93
and language production, 160–162
motor areas and, 111–112
orienting attention and, 133–137
safety, 59, 61–63
temporal resolution, 127
visual system and, 78
Restorative facilitation, 152, 155
Retina, 33
Retinal blindness. *See* Blindness
Reverse engineering, 3
Reversible deactivation techniques, 9. *See also* Lesions

Saccadic-onset latency, 106–108
Safety, 59–62
Sciatic nerve, 33, 35
Scientific theories and experiments, 11–12, 14

Search tasks. *See* Visual search tasks
Seizures, *See* Epileptic seizures
Sensorimotor cortex, 182
Sensory cortex, 165
Serial reaction-time test (SRTT), 185, 186, 194
Signal detection analysis, 66
Silent periods, 79–80
Single-pulse methodology, 76, 79, 83, 94–126
Single-pulse TMS, 5, 59. *See also specific topics*
Single-pulse TMS times, temporal window of, 79
Single-unit responses, latencies of, 77
Skill acquisition, 166, 184, 186–187, 193
Somatosensory cortex, 114, 153, 173, 176, 178–179, 181–183
Space-time, experimental, 5–8
Spatial and functional specificity of TMS, 53
Spatial effects in TMS, subtraction of, 57–58
Spatial processing, 105–106
Spatial resolution of TMS, xvi, 2, 3, 6, 7, 58, 96. *See also* Focality
Specificity. *See* Focality; Spatial resolution; Temporal resolution functional (*see* Cognitive resolution)
"Specter of compensation," 140
Speech arrest, 50, 157–159
Speech disorders, 199–200
Speech production, 83–84, 209. *See also* Language
Speed-accuracy trade-offs, 86
Speed of response. *See* Facilitations
Sprague effect, 152

Staining method, Golgi's, 12

Stimulation
  depth of, 56–58
  high vs. low rates of, 78–79
  low-frequency, 195
  simultaneous bilateral, 75–76
  sites of, 81–83

Stimulation mapping, electrical, 158

Stimulation parameters, 70–79

Striate cortex, 149, 183 See also visual areas
    and visual cortex

Superior colliculus, 152

Supplementary motor area (SMA), 53,
    111–112, 173

Supramarginal gyrus (SMG), 133, 135–137,
    139, 140

Tactile-detection tasks, 77, 114, 116, 155,
    211. See also Braille reading

Tactile discrimination, 177, 178

Tactile performance in the blind, 176–178

Tactile stimulation, 176

Tactile thresholds, 86

"Tan," 199

"Target present" and "target absent"
    responses. See Visual search tasks

Task analyses, x–xi

Temporal asynchrony in perception,
    123, 125

Temporal interactions between areas, 224

Temporal resolution of TMS, 2, 6, 7, 59, 79,
    96, 127–128

Temporo-parieto-occipital junction (TPO),
    75, 76

TEO, 148

Time. See also Temporal asynchrony
  sampling of, 76–79

Time lines, experimental, 89

Touch. See Tactile-detection tasks

Transcranial doppler sonography
    (TCD), 62

Transcranial magnetic stimulation (TMS),
    xii–xv, xvii, 4, 5, 8, 9, 14, 38, 50, 51, 54,
    55. See also specific topics
  applied prior to task, 131
  current era of, 39–43
  depth of penetration, 56–58
  discovering the mechanisms
    of, 28–38
  disruptive and productive modes, 45
  excitatory and inhibitory effects, 45
  first report of modern, 38
  functional localization, 54
  historical perspective on, 14
  secondary effects, 51
  sequence and time course of events in,
    39–43
  spatial modes of, 94 (see also specific modes)
  technical and ethical aspects, 4
  therapeutic, 214, 216–217
  therapeutic applications, 17
  TMS times, 69

Trigrams, 97–99

University of Sheffield, 36

Virtual-lesion effects, 111, 125

Virtual-lesion technique, 97

Virtual lesions, xv, 4, 93, 94, 205
  defined, 68, 69
  double, 93
  nature of, 65–69
  reversibility of, 8–9
Virtual patients, xv, 4
  creating, 65–94
  future of, 93–94
  types of, 93, 94
Visual areas
  V1, 7–8, 92, 99, 121, 123–125, 131, 148
    back projections to, 99
    necessity in visual imagery, 7–8
    orientation columns in, 82–83
  V4, 116, 121, 148
  V5/MT, 58, 70–75, 88, 121, 123, 124, 143,
    146–148, 153, 154, 187, 193
Visual binding, 100, 102, 106, 147
Visual cortex, 35, 50, 116, 177
  excitability, 204
  extrastriate, 125
  primary (*see* Visual areas, V1)
Visual masking, 97–99. *See also* Masking
    paradigm
Visual-orienting task. *See* Orienting
    attention
Visual search, 77, 82, 95, 100, 141, 142
Visual search tasks, 66, 101, 186–187
  conjunction search tasks, 100–105, 141,
    143, 144, 146
  PPC and, 82, 100, 102–106, 141–143, 145
Visual suppression curves, 97–99
Visual system, 116. *See also* Imagery
  effects of TMS in, 78

Visual-to-motor information
    processing, 116
Visuomotor association learning, 78
Visuomotor interaction, interhemispheric,
    86–88
Visuomotor learning, 73, 91

WADA test, 157
Wernicke's area, 159
Words and pseudowords, production of,
    160–162